Heart Failure and Palliative Care

A team approach

Edited by

Miriam Johnson

Senior Lecturer in Palliative Medicine
Hull York Medical School

and

Richard Lehman

General Practitioner
Banbury, Oxfordshire

Foreword by

Robert Twycross

Emeritus Clinical Reader in Palliative Medicine
Oxford University

Radcliffe Publishing
Oxford • Seattle

Radcliffe Publishing Ltd
18 Marcham Road
Abingdon
Oxon OX14 1AA
United Kingdom

www.radcliffe-oxford.com
Electronic catalogue and worldwide online ordering facility.

New research and clinical experience can result in changes in treatment and drug therapy. Readers of this book should therefore check the most recent product information on any drug they may prescribe to ensure they are complying with the manufacturer's recommendations concerning dosage, the method and duration of administration, and contraindications. Neither the publisher nor the authors accept liability for any injury or damage arising from this publication.

British Library Cataloguing in Publication Data

A catalogue record for this book is available from the British Library.

ISBN-10: 1 85775 643 6
ISBN-13: 978 1 85775 643 2

Typeset by Ann Buchan (Typesetters), Middlesex
Printed and bound by TJ International, Padstow, Cornwall

Contents

Foreword   iv
Preface   vi
About the editors   viii
List of contributors   ix
Acknowledgements   x

1 **The need for palliative care in heart failure**   1
   Richard Lehman

2 **The syndrome of advanced heart failure**   20
   Richard Lehman

3 **Maximum therapy for heart failure**   31
   Michael Davies

4 **Prognosis in advanced heart failure**   44
   Richard Lehman

5 **Symptom relief for advanced heart failure**   60
   Miriam Johnson and Louise Gibbs

6 **Supportive care: psychological, social and spiritual aspects**   74
   Scott Murray, Marilyn Kendall, Richard Lehman and Miriam Johnson

7 **Communication in heart failure**   87
   Iain Lawrie and Suzanne Kite

8 **Care of the patient dying from heart failure**   110
   Clare Littlewood and Miriam Johnson

9 **Palliative care needs of young people with heart failure**   119
   Hayley Pryse-Hawkins

10 **Palliative care services for patients with heart failure**   134
   Miriam Johnson with contributions from Andrew Daley, Clare Littlewood,
   Jo Sykes, Tim Chester and Dorothy McElroy

   Index   144

Foreword

Thirty years ago, palliative care generally implied inpatient terminal care for cancer patients. Since then, the term has gradually expanded to describe a concept of care with its own defining characteristics which is applicable to all forms of end-stage disease, and which is delivered as much in the community as in a hospice or hospital. However, despite the broader definition, much remains to be done to turn health theory and policy into universally available practice. That is why this book is both necessary and timely. To quote one of the editors:

> *'Palliative care for heart failure is now on the map, but much of the detail of the map has yet to be drawn.'*

Heart Failure and Palliative Care: a team approach is an exciting book. It is exciting for the traditional 'old-style' palliative care clinician (like me) whose practice and expertise is almost entirely limited to end-stage malignant disease. I believe it will also be exciting for cardiology clinicians. It will liberate them (if liberation is needed) from the narrow 'biomedical' model of disease management and enable them to adopt a more holistic patient-centred approach. This means that the focus will be on a *person* with heart failure, rather than a person with *heart failure*. On paper this may seem a small difference, but in practice the change of focus has a big effect.

The key to success is *good communication* between the health professionals on the one hand, and the patient and family on the other. Indeed, palliative care should be seen as *a partnership between experts*. In relation to the disease process, the clinicians are the experts, but in relation to the impact of the illness, the experts are the patient and family. It is vital to recognise this because, through listening to their story and their problems, the patient and family begin to shift from being passive victims to empowered persons. For demoralised patients, both speed and time is of the essence. As one patient is reported as saying:

> *I am pleased how quickly you responded to the referral from my cardiologist, and pleased at the length of time you were prepared to sit and listen to my problems and work out solutions. The follow-up from the district nurse was also very prompt.*

Generally speaking, a short prognosis is the entry ticket to specific palliative care services. However, prognostication is not as straightforward in progressive heart failure as it is with most patients with advanced cancer. Fortunately, this book shows that there is a pragmatic way forward through the morass of uncertainties, and that is to ask the 'surprise question'. *'Would I be surprised if this patient died within the next year?'* If the answer is 'No', then it is time to adopt a palliative approach to care. Paradoxically, despite its seemingly unscientific nature, the question is in fact the only scientifically acceptable one in this context, and provides a satisfactory basis for a proactive change in the overall direction of care.

One of the many things in this book that excited me was learning about specialist heart failure nurses. Such nurses are clearly the crucial link between cardiology and palliative care. Here is someone who could ensure that I was up to date with current cardiological prescribing practice, and, equally, who could ensure that, when indicated, heart failure patients were seamlessly referred for specific palliative care. Further, given the needs of the families, it occurred to me that if heart failure patients were able to attend the local palliative care day centre, it would be a good way for established palliative care services to become more involved – given the active support of the local heart failure nurse.

However, to care optimally for patients with end-stage heart failure, palliative care specialists will need to develop a novel-for-them approach to care. For example, cancer patients receiving chemotherapy often feel worse for their anticancer treatment, and the default position in palliative care is to encourage its discontinuation if the burdens of treatment appear to outweigh any benefits. In contrast, the patient with heart failure generally feels better for disease-specific treatment, and it needs to be continued, judiciously adjusted, perhaps simplified, and closely monitored. Further, palliative care in heart failure could be intimidating because of the need to enter a Brave New World littered with interventions which may significantly improve the patient's physical status, and even prognosis – a world which includes CRT, ICD, LVAD, CPR and even heart transplantation. But here again, with the support and advice of the heart failure nurse in particular, it should be possible for palliative care specialists to successfully negotiate their way through this minefield of additional treatment possibilities.

The corresponding challenge for cardiologists is to make sure that their most needy patients do not miss out on the added benefits of a palliative approach to care. The most needy patients will include those who are being considered for a 'high-tech' intervention. But it is these who perhaps are least likely to be referred to a palliative care service because 'We're not at that stage yet – there's still a lot more we can do'. In consequence, the myriad other problems contributing to the patient's misery fester unaddressed on the sidelines.

The 20th century was a time of unparalleled, and at times incredible, advances in medical science and the treatment of disease. Let us hope that the 21st century will be the time when medicine generally becomes truly holistic, with close attention to the whole person, rather than just to the disease process. Although much still needs to be done, there is definitely light at the end of the tunnel. The day is dawning when it will no longer be true that 'you've got to have cancer to get good palliative care'.

Robert Twycross DM, FRCP
Emeritus Clinical Reader in Palliative Medicine
Oxford University
June 2006

Preface

'Think for a month, write for an hour' is advice sometimes given to those who want to add to the medical literature. The contributors to this book have each been thinking about palliative care and heart failure for years. Each of us felt that it was time to put something on paper. This is not, then, one of those books which distils a well-established body of knowledge, still less does it attempt to be 'definitive'. Rather, it is an attempt to bring together the knowledge and experience of a wide range of professionals to create a framework for looking at and addressing the needs of those dying from heart failure. It is an exercise in joined-up thinking, across boundaries of professional group and medical specialty, in an attempt to create a framework that we hope more and more people can build on over time. We have tried wherever possible to be evidence based, but the evidence base for many areas, particularly symptom control and service provision, is sadly lacking. Out of the gaps we hope will emerge a research agenda for palliative care in heart failure.

Palliative care for heart failure involves a huge potential range of expertise, and to keep up with its literature requires the scanning of journals in social science, psychology, general medicine, geriatric medicine, nursing, rehabilitation, spiritual care, palliative care, primary care, and both general and specialist cardiology. In all this, it is all too easy to forget the people who are actually living through the distressing and difficult end-stage of heart failure – patients and their families. The only prize they seek is relief from distress and a peaceful death. This is not a theoretical subject and this book is not in any way an academic exercise. It is time to listen to the voices of those who suffer, time to think outside our own particular field of expertise. It is time to work together with others who can add so much more to the care of these patients, whose disease affects every domain of life.

This book is therefore written by doctors and nurses who are clinicians first and academics only second, if at all. One of the editors achieved brief fame as a Sheffield teenager in the guise of 'City Rocket Youth', when he and a friend attempted to build a crude rocket in the school metalwork department. Looking after end-stage heart failure is not rocket science. It is much more difficult. The trajectory of a rocket is predictable: the course of heart failure is not. Patients are not made of metal, and it matters what happens to them.

At the same time we do not want to overemphasise the complexities of the subject. Simple things may be what patients need most. We will know that our efforts – and those of many others – have succeeded when palliative care for heart failure is no longer a novel idea but an assumed part of routine care. This will certainly require leadership and innovation on a wide scale, and it is encouraging to see how this is already happening. It will also involve a gradual change of attitude, brought about by educational programmes in primary care and at a basic level of secondary care. Palliative care for cancer has become a routine part of general practice and community nursing, and it should not be too daunting a task to extend this to heart failure. Similarly, the junior doctors and general medical ward staff who admit patients with heart failure need to be encouraged to look for help from liaison palliative care services and to apply an end-of-life care pathway when appropriate.

This book started from plans to set up an interactive website, which we hope may yet happen. However, even in the electronic age of knowledge, a book can form a nucleus around which others can develop their ideas, in a way that a website would be unlikely to achieve. We hope that those reading this book will be inspired to look at local ways to address the inequity of access to supportive and palliative care for patients with heart failure. We hope that a future book might describe a very different picture as the research base of symptom control and service provision develops over coming years.

Miriam Johnson
Richard Lehman
June 2006

About the editors

Dr Miriam Johnson graduated in 1984, three years before palliative medicine became a specialty in the UK. She trained in general practice and then spent some years in haematology before entering higher specialist training in palliative medicine in the west of Scotland, completing in 1999. During her specialist registrar training she completed her MD thesis, 'Venous thromboembolism and advanced cancer', and developed her interest in the palliative care of heart failure patients. She is also a 'Regional Champion' for the Liverpool Care Pathway.

The interest in heart failure has grown since her appointment as consultant palliative physician to St Catherine's Hospice, Scarborough, where she has developed one of the first UK joint services for heart failure patients between palliative care and cardiology colleagues. She is also lead palliative physician for the Humber and Yorkshire Coast Cancer Network.

In April 2006 she took up a senior lectureship in palliative medicine with the Hull York Medical School, where she hopes to develop her research and teaching interests.

Dr Richard Lehman has had an interest in palliative care since becoming a general practitioner at Hightown Surgery in Banbury, Oxfordshire, in 1979. Following the death of his father from heart failure in 1991, he has developed a special interest in the promotion of palliative care for patients with advanced heart failure. He has also published research and comment on the use of B-type natriuretic peptide in heart failure in primary care. He is a senior research fellow at the Department of Primary Medical Care in the University of Oxford.

However, he remains a nearly full-time GP and a generalist at heart, contributing regular reviews of the general medical literature to the *BMJ* website, *Evidence-Based Medicine* and the Doctors.Net website. His other interests are in student teaching and the medical humanities.

List of contributors

Tim Chester
Heart Failure Nurse Specialist, Torbay Hospital, South Devon Healthcare Trust, Torquay, Devon

Andrew Daley
Consultant Palliative Physician, Marie Curie Hospice, Bradford

Michael Davies
Consultant Cardiologist, Selly Oak Hospital, Birmingham

Louise Gibbs
Consultant Palliative Physician, St Christopher's Hospice, Sydenham

Miriam Johnson
Senior Lecturer in Palliative Medicine, Hull York Medical School; Consultant Palliative Physician, St Catherine's Hospice, Scarborough

Marilyn Kendall
Research Fellow, Primary Palliative Care Research Group, Division of Community Health Sciences; General Practice, University of Edinburgh

Suzanne Kite
Consultant in Palliative Medicine, Palliative Care Team, Leeds Teaching Hospitals NHS Trust (LGI)

Iain Lawrie
Specialist Registrar in Palliative Medicine, Yorkshire Palliative Medicine Training Scheme, Leeds Teaching Hospitals NHS Trust

Richard Lehman
General Practitioner, Banbury, Oxon

Clare Littlewood
Macmillan Consultant in Palliative Medicine, St Helens and Knowsley Hospitals, Willowbrook Hospice, Merseyside

Dorothy McElroy
Ardgowan Hospice, Greenock, Strathclyde

Scott Murray
St Columba's Hospice Professor of Primary Palliative Care, Primary Palliative Care Research Group; General Practice, University of Edinburgh

Hayley Pryse-Hawkins
Heart Failure Nurse, Royal Brompton and Harefield NHS Trust; BHF Nurse Coordinator

Jo Sykes
Consultant Palliative Physician, Torbay Hospital, South Devon Healthcare Trust, Torquay, Devon

Acknowledgements

We would like to thank all our chapter authors for their contributions, which in every case involved the hard work of breaking new ground and making new connections. We are also very grateful for the support and help of many other individuals who have encouraged us in this project, especially Robert Twycross, Michael Connolly, Christopher Ward and Peter Tebbit. Bringing the book together has involved time and effort, which inevitably have been taken away from other activities, and we are grateful to our work colleagues for their kindness and understanding on occasions when this has been apparent. Finally, we would like to thank our spouses for their patience and support, without which this book could not have been completed.

Miriam Johnson
Richard Lehman

Chapter 1

The need for palliative care in heart failure

Richard Lehman

More than 40 years ago, John Hinton conducted a study at King's College Hospital in London, which examined – for the first time ever in a structured way – the physical and mental distress of patients dying on the medical ward of an acute hospital. Most of the patients had cancer, but there was also a group of 14 who were dying of heart or renal failure. This study[1] proved a major stimulus to the development of 'terminal care', as it was then known, and to the growth of the hospice movement in Great Britain. Terminal care in the UK grew up in most places as a voluntary provision, centred around an inpatient facility, which, if it existed at all, was usually precariously maintained by charitable funding. Many of the charities that supported hospices or home care for the dying were specifically cancer charities, and as a result many hospices restricted their services to the care of patients dying of cancer. To a considerable extent, this tradition still influences the provision of palliative services in the UK.

Throughout the world, the literature of palliative care has become a very rich literature about the relief of physical, mental, social and spiritual distress in people dying from disseminated cancer. There is much less about dying from other causes, with the possible exception of AIDS. But those who pioneered terminal care did not start with such a narrow focus. If we return to the Hinton study, we find him observing that: 'Discomfort was not necessarily greatest in those dying from cancer; patients dying of heart failure, or renal failure, or both, had most physical distress.' Many of the features described in later studies were already carefully set down in this paper – the greater predominance of dyspnoea and nausea, and the anxiety and depression associated with the long and unpredictable course of progressive heart failure.

Historically, then, the needs have long been known, but has it taken until the last few years for this large area of neglected distress to be recognised and addressed.

Part One: The experience of advanced heart failure

Patient voices

> *'I want to be treated like a human being, not a lump of flesh everyone is trying to get rid of.' Mr E*

Dying from heart failure can be a very prolonged and difficult process. It often involves exhaustion and uncertainty for both patient and carers. Over the past decade, several studies have recorded and analysed the experience of patients with a diagnosis of heart failure. The most general and accessible for teaching purposes is in the Database of Individual Patient Experiences (DIPEx; www.dipex.org/heartfailure). This contains interviews carried out in 2004 with 42 patients selected to represent a wide range of people with all grades of heart failure.

The earliest studies to explore the experience of heart failure patients in detail were carried out in the UK and New Zealand in 1998–9. In Auckland, New Zealand, Stephen Buetow and colleagues carried out interviews with 62 heart failure patients in the community.[2] Some of their findings about coping strategies[3] are discussed in Chapter 6. One striking finding of their study is that many patients with heart failure do not have any useful understanding of their diagnosis. This lack of understanding also featured in a hospital-based study carried out by Angie Rogers and colleagues in London.[4] They also uncovered a wide range of symptoms, discussed in the next section.

The most detailed study to look specifically at patients with advanced heart failure was carried out in Edinburgh, and published in 2002.[5] Marilyn Kendall carried out 219 interviews with 40 patients with heart failure or lung cancer, together with their main carer, every three months for up to one year. This study gives us valuable insights into the differences between the two conditions (*see* below), but above all into the unalleviated misery experienced by many of the heart failure patients and those closest to them. This study is discussed more fully in Chapter 6. It contains many telling quotes, some of which are interspersed throughout this chapter. Here are a few others:

> *'I slipped down the bed and oh panic attacks I got, and I had to sit up, I couldn't get my breath. I felt, oh I can't really, you can't actually tell people.'* Mr HH

> *'You can't do what you did before, things you took for granted are now an impossible dream, I feel useless.'* Mr K

> *'There's not an awful lot we can do for people like him.'* GP of Mr T

> *'I think he probably needs a gun… if you were a horse, they would shoot you.'* Carer of Mr N

Problems and symptoms

> *'The sickness makes me fell lousy. I'm taking that many tablets now and I don't know what's the reaction. You sort one thing out and it starts another.'* Mr E

Heart failure is a syndrome that can affect every organ in the body, in ways that are outlined in the next chapter. Also, as the quotation above illustrates, treatments used for heart failure often bring their own symptoms, such as polyuria, hypotension, tiredness or cough. The symptoms of heart failure have been assessed and quantified in a number of studies at various stages of the condition. Here is a list of the (predominantly physical) symptoms found by Rogers in the qualitative study previously mentioned:[4]

Breathlessness	21 (77%)
Tiredness	16 (59%)
Chest pain	13 (48%)
Joint pain	14 (52%)
Poor sleep	16 (59%)
Feeling down	13 (48%)
Confusion/short-term memory loss	12 (44%)
Dizziness	6 (22%)
Loss of appetite	6 (22%)

The patients in this study were mostly unable to distinguish whether these symptoms were caused by heart failure, their treatment or another condition. This is a daunting list, but other studies have produced even longer ones.[6–8] We also need to remember that other problems may be even more important to the patients and to the carers – such things as social isolation, constant uncertainty and loss of the will to live. Palliative care for heart failure needs to address a range of physical, social, psychological and spiritual issues which can be even wider than in most cancers.

Loss of quality of life is a feature of heart failure in all of its stages. As part of a general survey of the epidemiology of heart failure in the West Midlands,[9] Richard Hobbs and colleagues measured the overall effect of heart failure due to systolic dysfunction, using the SF36 questionnaire. In all domains, patients with heart failure of any cause scored markedly lower than the general population, and in most domains lower than those with other chronic illnesses, mental or physical (Figure 1.1).

Looking specifically at the last six months of life, we have evidence from studies in three different countries that the symptom burden increases steadily. A common feature of all these studies is that pain is a frequent and severe symptom in many heart failure patients who are near to death. In the SUPPORT study,[7] carried out in a number of US academic medical centres during the 1990s, 41% of patients

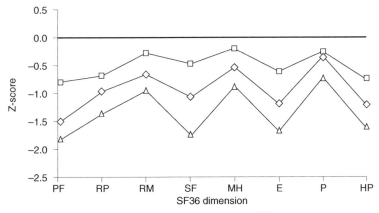

Z-scores of diagnosed heart failure patients divided into NYHA classes compared to the general population. PF=physical functioning; RP= role physical; RM= role mental; SF= social functioning; MH= mental health; E= energy; P=pain; HP= overall perception of health; —— = general population; □=NYHA class II; ◇ =NYHA class III; △=NYHA class IV.

Figure 1.1 Quality of life in heart failure. By permission of Oxford University Press from Hobbs *et al.* (2002).[9]

were reportedly in pain in the three days before death. A Swedish study carried out at the same time[8] produced similar findings, and commented that although numerous distressing symptoms were well documented by doctors and nurses, there was little evidence that they were being adequately addressed.

Several other studies have looked in different ways at the symptom burden of heart failure in all its stages and the way it affects quality of life. These illustrate that supportive care, in the sense of good communication and a holistic approach, is needed from the time of first diagnosis of heart failure. As the condition progresses, palliative care in its traditional role becomes increasingly important. In an ideal world, there would be no distinction between supportive and palliative care, and one would grade imperceptibly into the other. This ideal is still some way from being achieved in cancer, and in heart failure the task has scarcely begun.

The illness trajectory

> 'One day I'll be on top, the next day back under again.' Mr R

A typical feature of heart failure is fluctuation between periods of what are referred to as compensation and decompensation. The aim of treatment in heart failure is to compensate for reduced cardiac output by damping down the adverse neurohormonal effects which it produces, and reducing fluid overload. The resulting physiological equilibrium allows a degree of steady function, albeit at an impaired level. When this equilibrium breaks down, decompensation results and the patient becomes distressed, with breathlessness and/or increasing oedema. As we saw in one of quotes above, the experience of near drowning can be terrifying, and it often results in hospital admission. In most developed countries, decompensated heart failure is now the commonest cause of acute medical admission.

This process can be depicted in a disease trajectory diagram which looks like a downward slope interrupted by a number of sharp dips, in contrast with the trajectories of cancer and general frailty (Figure 1.2).[10]

This kind of diagrammatic representation is very useful for teaching purposes, but it has its limitations. Most published studies have concentrated on the physical disease trajectory of heart failure without dealing with social, psychological or spiritual trajectories. In reality, separate aspects of the patient experience may follow different trajectories. For example, the psychological effect of a first decompensation may be even more marked than the physical effects, resulting in long-term anxiety; or a spiritual trajectory of increasing acceptance may occur at the same time as physical decline. No two patients will follow exactly the same trajectory in each of these aspects.

In the past, many have seen the unpredictability of heart failure as an obstacle to palliative care deployment. In cancer, there is a definite moment when incurable spread is discovered and the focus shifts to symptom control, but there is no such defined point in heart failure. There is the additional problem that nearly half of all patients with heart failure will die suddenly, and only a proportion of these will show any warning signs of deterioration. Taking a narrow and pessimistic view of the meaning of palliative care, it could be argued that there

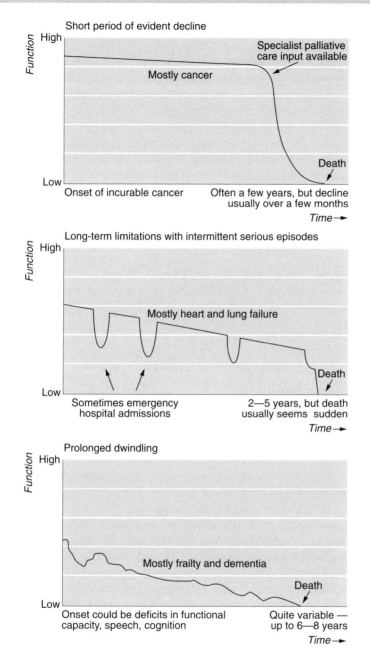

Figure 1.2 Schematic disease trajectories. With permission of the BMJ and the RAND Corporation from Murray *et al.* (2005).[10]

is simply no way to deploy it in a timely and cost-effective manner when the disease process is so unpredictable.[11] We shall argue strongly against this position throughout this book. For now we will simply state that the prognostic uncertainty of heart failure is not as great as it might first appear (*see* Chapter 4), and most palliative care professionals are now moving away from the model of terminal care for the incurable towards a model of supportive care for everyone with a life-shortening illness.

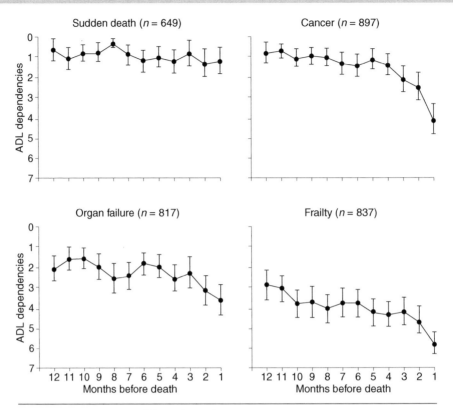

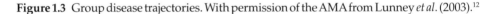

Error bars indicate 95% confidence intervals.

Figure 1.3 Group disease trajectories. With permission of the AMA from Lunney *et al.* (2003).[12]

The typical disease trajectory for cancer was drawn very differently from that of heart failure in the schematic diagram of Figure 1.2. However, in studies of whole patient groups, these differences may less extreme (Figure 1.3).[12]

This does not negate the heart failure trajectory as shown above, because it depicts only the mean group disability for various types of organ failure. The trajectory in individuals can be much more labile, particularly in heart failure, but also in some types of cancer. For example, patients with haematological cancers can alternate between near-normal health and periods of severe morbidity due to chemotherapy or neutropenic fever. In the next section we shall look at some comparisons between heart failure and cancer.

Heart failure and cancer compared

There are some striking similarities between the characteristics of heart failure patients and the elderly cancer patients who already form the bulk of the palliative care caseload. McKinley and colleagues looked at the records of 154 patients in two general practices in Leicester who died between 2000 and 2002.[13] Of these, 108 died of cancer and 46 of cardiorespiratory disease. In both groups, the average age at death was 74, and there was no significant difference in the number of co-morbidities.

Table 1.1 Palliative care clinic and heart failure clinic compared: analysis of most troublesome problems

	Palliative care (n = 213)	Heart failure (n = 66)
Physical	346 (57)	34 (20)
Cardiac	–	99 (58)
Social/functional	199 (33)	23 (14)
Psychiatric	59 (10)	14 (8)
Total number of problems	604	170
Problem	Number of patients (%)	Number of patients (%)
Pain/angina	104 (49)	21 (32)
Loss of independence	64 (30)	13 (20)
Difficulty walking	58 (27)	15 (23)
Anxiety or depression	47 (22)	10 (15)
Tiredness	40 (19)	18 (27)
Breathlessness	38 (18)	36 (55)
Constipation	32 (15)	2 (3)
Nausea or vomiting	28 (13)	3 (5)
Difficulty sleeping	11 (5)	7 (11)

Source: With permission of Edward Arnold (Publishers) Ltd from Anderson *et al.*[6]

Looking at the issues from a hospital perspective, an important study was carried out by Heather Anderson and colleagues in 1996,[6] based around the first hospital clinic in the UK specifically for heart failure, set up by Christopher Ward in Manchester. This compared the needs expressed by patients attending the heart failure clinic and those receiving palliative care for cancer. Usefully, this study not only lists the symptoms experienced by the two groups of patients, but also compares those that were perceived as most troublesome (Table 1.1).

In the Edinburgh study cited above,[5] from which we have taken our patient quotations, Murray and Kendall provide a wide-ranging comparative analysis of the main themes from interviews with sufferers from lung cancer and from heart failure (Table 1.2).

These studies and others[14] show that although the relative severity of symptoms can differ between heart failure and cancer, the total symptom load is certainly no lighter and may often be greater. Studies carried out a decade ago also reached the conclusion that the provision of symptom relief for cancer patients was much better than for heart failure. Although the situation is changing, this still remains true for the vast majority of patients.

Prognosis of heart failure and common cancers

Heart failure has often been referred to as a 'malignant' disease, with a prognosis worse than that of several disseminated cancers. This was strikingly demonstrated in a study by Simon Stewart and colleagues, who analysed data from all first hospital admissions in 1991 in Scotland for the commonest cancers and heart failure.[15] The Scottish Morbidity Record Scheme was used to trace patients and calculate the five-year survival for each cancer and for heart failure following first admission.

Table 1.2 Summary comparison of the experience of patients having lung cancer and heart failure

Lung cancer	Heart failure
• Cancer trajectory with clearer terminal phase. Able to plan for death	• Gradual decline punctuated by episodes of acute deterioration. Sudden, usually unexpected, death with no distinct terminal phase
• Good understanding of diagnosis and prognosis	• Little understanding of diagnosis and prognosis
• 'How long have I got?'	• 'I know it won't get better, but I hope it won't get any worse'
• Swinging between hope and despair	• Daily grind of hopelessness
• Lung cancer takes over life and becomes overriding concern	• Much co-morbidity to cope with; heart often not seen as main issue
• Treatment calendar dominates life; more contact with services and professionals	• Shrinking social world dominates life, little contact with health and social services
• Feel worse on treatment: coping with side effects	• Feel better on treatment: work of balancing and monitoring in the community
• Relatives anxious	• Relatives isolated and exhausted
• Financial benefits accessible	• Less access to benefits with uncertain prognosis
• Specialist services often available in the community	• Specialist services rarely available in the community
• Care prioritised early as 'cancer', and later as 'terminally ill'	• Less priority as a 'chronic disease', and less priority later as uncertain if yet 'terminally ill'

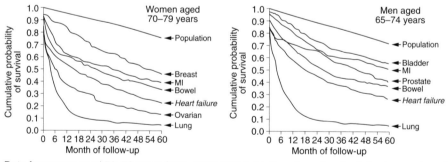

Data for women aged 70–79 years (28% of the total cohort) are based on the following number of patients: heart failure ($n = 1167$), myocardial infarction ($n = 1600$) and cancer of the lung ($n = 475$), breast ($n = 441$), bowel ($n = 369$) and ovary ($n = 108$). Similarly data for men aged 65–74 years (26% of the total cohort) are based on the following numbers of patients: heart failure ($n = 1063$), myocardial infarction ($n = 2083$) and cancer of the lung ($n = 1064$), bowel ($n = 485$), prostate ($n = 452$) and bladder ($n = 264$).

Figure 1.4 Age-specific probability of survival following a first admission for heart failure, myocardial infarction and the four most common types of cancer specific to men and women relative to the overall population. With permission of the European Society of Cardiology from Stewart *et al.* (2001).[15]

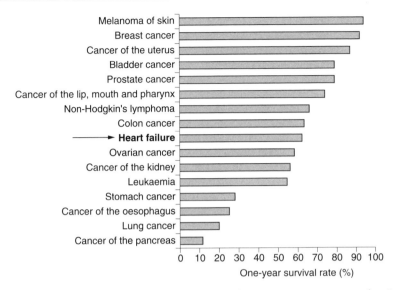

Figure 1.5 One-year survival rates, heart failure and major cancers compared, mid-1990s, England and Wales. From Cowie *et al.* (2000).[16] www.heartstats.org

Similar results have been obtained by comparing the survival of patients with incident heart failure in the Hillingdon study[16] with the survival rates for major cancers provided by the Office for National Statistics for England and Wales (Figure 1.5).

Much depends on the staging of each cancer, and on how one chooses to define 'heart failure'. It is probably true that prognostic variability in heart failure is also greater. But Scott Murray has rightly warned of the danger of 'prognostic paralysis'[17] resulting from too much concern about predictability: the main message here is that by the time a heart failure patient has required hospital admission, the risk of death in the next 18 months is over 40%.

Co-morbidity

'It' just one thing after another, really. Which illness shall I start with?' Ms I

'The heart problem doesn't seem to be the thing that bothers us. The other illnesses are so obvious that her heart didn't enter the equation.' Carer of Mrs LL

Any patient with heart failure inevitably has co-morbidity, because 'heart failure' is not a diagnosis but the label used to describe the result of a disease process affecting the body's capacity to maintain an adequate circulation. The commonest disease processes are ischaemic heart disease, diabetes and/or long-standing hypertension, and 90% patients with heart failure have one or more of these. The heart failure syndrome can in turn lead to other co-morbidities, such as depression, cognitive impairment or renal failure. Lastly, since heart failure is mostly a disease of old age, patients often have a number of unconnected health problems, such as cancer, osteoarthritis, hearing difficulty, macular degeneration and so on.

Table 1.3 Twenty most common non-cardiac chronic disease conditions for patients age ≥ 65 years with coronary heart disease (*n* = 122,630). With permission of the American College of Cardiology Foundation from Braunstein *et al.*[19]

Chronic disease defined by CCS code	% Prevalence (n)
Essential hypertension	55 (67,211)
Diabetes mellitus	31 (38,175)
COPD and bronchiectasis	26 (32,275)
Ocular disorders (retinopathy, macular disease, cataract, glaucoma)	24 (29,548)
Hypercholesterolaemia	21 (25,219)
Peripheral and visceral atherosclerosis	16 (20,027)
Osteoarthritis	16 (19,929)
Chronic respiratory failure/insufficiency/ arrest or other lower respiratory disease excluding COPD/bronchiectasis	14 (17,610)
Thyroid disorders	14 (16,751)
Hypertension with complications and secondary hypertension	11 (13,732)
Alzheimer's disease/dementia	9 (10,839)
Depression/affective disorders	8 (9,371)
Chronic renal failure	7 (8,652)
Prostatic hyperplasia	7 (8,077)
Intravertebral injury, spondylosis or other chronic back disorders	7 (8,469)
Asthma	5 (6,717)
Osteoporosis	5 (6,688)
Renal insufficiency (acute and unspecified renal failure)	4 (5,259)
Anxiety, somatoform disorders, and personality disorders	3 (3,978)
Cerebrovascular disease, late effects	3 (3,750)

CCS = Clinical Classification System; CHF = chronic heart failure; COPD = chronic obstructive pulmonary disease.

Thus the words 'co-morbidity' or 'concomitant disorder' can be used in three ways in heart failure:

- to describe conditions which play a causal role in heart failure
- to describe the secondary effects of the heart failure itself
- to describe unrelated health problems.

Most, but not all, studies[12] have found that heart failure patients have a greater burden of co-morbidity than cancer patients.[18] Table 1.3 shows the co-morbidities in a large US heart failure cohort study.[19]

The high prevalence of co-morbidity in heart failure, like the wide range of the symptom burden, means that co-ordinated team effort is required to address the needs of most patients. The specialties with greatest expertise in this are primary care, palliative care and gerontology or general medicine, rather than cardiology. Most cardiologists are aware of this.[20] There is no place for tunnel vision in the management of advanced heart failure and its many associated illnesses.

Part Two: Assessing palliative care need

The size of the problem

When the need for palliative care in heart failure became the subject of correspondence in the general medical journals 10 or more years ago,[21,22] a frequently expressed anxiety was that this would 'open the floodgates' and overwhelm specialist palliative care services. At first sight, the epidemiology of heart failure appears to confirm this fear: a recent European survey suggests that nearly one person in three will suffer from heart failure at some stage.[23] Fortunately, this has not been the experience of those palliative care services brave enough to have lowered their flood defences (*see* Chapter 10). As in so much else to do with heart failure, there are clearly complex factors at work.

It is difficult to work out the likely load on specialist and other palliative care services from the available data, but we will begin by taking the approach set out by Tebbit for the population-based needs assessment in the palliative care of cancer.[24] This is a very useful framework for establishing comparative levels of need in specific locations: it is not intended to reach conclusions about absolute levels of service requirement. Tebbit suggests three elements in estimating service need: epidemiological, demographic and socioeconomic.

Epidemiological approach

The epidemiology of 'heart failure' is often difficult to interpret because there is no clear, universally agreed definition of heart failure that can be applied to all population studies. This contrasts sharply with cancer, where there is almost always a firmly established tissue diagnosis. However, by the time heart failure has reached class III and IV of the New York Heart Association (NYHA) classification, there is usually little difficulty in recognising it as a clinical syndrome (Box 1.1).

Box 1.1 NYHA classification of heart failure

Class I
No limitations. Ordinary physical activity does not cause fatigue, breathlessness or palpitation.

Class II
Slight limitation of physical activity. Comfortable at rest. Ordinary physical activity results in fatigue, palpitation, breathlessness or angina pectoris.

Class III
Marked limitation of physical activity. Although patients are comfortable at rest, less than ordinary activity will lead to symptoms.

Class IV
Inability to carry out any physical activity without discomfort. Symptoms of congestive cardiac failure are present even at rest. With any physical activity increased discomfort is experienced.

Table 1.4 Place and mode of death in two major interventional studies

Study	In hospital	Out of hospital	Not reported
AIRE			
Sudden	133	135	
Chronic heart failure	182	10	
Total	315	145	
UK, post-infarction only; 45% of pts who died suddenly had severe or worsening HF before death[28]			
ATLAS			
Sudden	149	439	1
Chronic heart failure	309	97	39
Other	271	71	7
Total	729	607	47
Multi-national, mixed aetiology[29]			

Estimates of the total prevalence of heart failure in the UK vary widely, between 0.5 and 3 million. The estimate reached in 2002 by the British Heart Foundation website is 878,000.[25] There are no UK epidemiological data on heart failure stratified by NHYA class, and the general quality of data relating to heart disease in the UK has been called into question by some epidemiologists.[26]

Mortality

Mortality from heart failure would seem relatively easy to establish, but this is not true for the UK and for many other countries that follow international guidelines on the certification of death. The preamble which advises doctors how to complete UK death certificates repeatedly warns against stating heart failure as a cause of death. According to international advice, heart failure is a mode rather than a cause of death. If this advice was followed to the letter, the UK would have no recorded deaths in which the primary cause was heart failure. This is also true of most countries that register death on the basis of a single underlying cause.[26]

There are two possible ways to get around this problem, especially when trying to estimate the local death rate from heart failure. One is to examine death certificates for *any* mention of heart failure, rather than looking only at conventional data on the underlying cause. This is the approach taken by Goldacre and colleagues in a study of the former Oxfordshire Region of the NHS.[27] This may be useful for detecting a trend, as in their study, which shows a decline in mortality from heart failure in line with the overall decline in cardiac disease. But it is still likely to provide a gross underestimate of the total number dying from heart failure.

The second approach relies on evidence that nearly all patients dying from progressive heart failure do so in hospital, whereas a greater proportion of heart failure patients who die suddenly do so outside hospital. Unfortunately the data are imprecise and variable, as can be seen in Table 1.4. In the UK study (AIRE[28]), fewer than a third of heart failure deaths occurred outside hospital, whereas in the international study (ATLAS[29]), the numbers were more equal.

This leaves us with very uncertain quantification of mortality for heart failure, in contrast with the well recorded data we have for specific cancers.

Mode and place of death

Death from heart failure can be sudden, due to electrical instability or a new ischaemic event, or slow, due to progressive organ failure and pulmonary oedema. All grades of heart failure carry an increased risk of sudden death, which usually happens outside hospital. Class IV heart failure (NYHA classification) is the terminal phase, and when such patients decompensate, their distress and breathlessness is such that they are almost always admitted to hospital. Studies of the mode and place of death in heart failure therefore show a division between sudden deaths predominantly outside hospital and death from progressive heart failure ('pump failure') predominantly within hospital (Table 1.4).

Demographic approach

This aspect of a needs assessment examines the age and sex structure of the population and extrapolates from the known epidemiology of the condition to reach an estimate of the likely disease burden. Again, major differences in the diagnostic criteria and the available data make this difficult (Table 1.5).

The wide variations in absolute percentages make it impossible at present to make useful predictions of service demand in specific localities, let alone the whole of the UK. Apart from the epidemiological uncertainties, it seems that social factors also play a major part in service use by heart failure patients (*see* socioeconomic section below).

Ethnicity

Ethnicity is an issue that has received much international attention in the study of heart failure,[31] even to the extent of recruiting specific ethnic groups to major interventional trials. Data from the UK, however, are scanty. Looking at ischaemic heart disease, which is the precursor of most systolic heart failure, there are wide variations between the main ethnic groups in England.[32] The lowest rates are found in the Chinese and Black Caribbean populations, the highest in the Pakistani and Bangladeshi groups.

Heart failure has been found to present at an earlier age in South Asian men in studies carried out in Leicester,[33] Birmingham[34] and Harrow.[35] These studies do not show conclusively that the overall prevalence of heart failure is greater in South Asian immigrant populations, although this is likely. It seems that in these groups, heart failure presents earlier and is associated with better survival.[36]

Living in households: the needs of carers

Most patients with advanced heart failure are elderly and live with a spouse on whom they become highly dependent. There are few data about the marital status of such patients, but the Manchester study[6] found that 82% were married and living with a spouse, a much higher percentage than their cancer cohort. The physical, mental and spiritual exhaustion that carers can suffer are well demonstrated in the narrative studies, as we saw in one of the quotes above ('if you were a horse, they would shoot you'). The needs of heart failure patients who do not have a family carer are even greater.[37]

Table 1.5 Studies of heart failure prevalence in the UK[30]

Source	Study	Year	Place	Men				Women			
				45–54 %	55–64 %	65–74 %	75–84 %	45–54 %	55–64 %	65–74 %	75–84 %
Royal College of General Practitioners et al. 1995	4th National Study of Morbidity Statistics from General Practice	1991/92	England and Wales		0.5*	3.2	8.0		0.4*	2.3	7.1
McDonagh et al. 1997	MONICA	1992	Glasgow		2.5	3.2			2.0	3.6	
Mair et al. 1996	Two general practices in Liverpool	1994	Liverpool		2.7	5.3	10.4**		1.2	5.1	13.3**
Office for National Statistics 2000	Key Health Statistics from General Practice	1998	England and Wales	0.3	1.4	4.5	10.9	0.2	0.9	3.6	9.9
Davies et al. 2001	Heart of England Screening Study	1995/99	West Midlands	0.3	2.7	4.2	7.3	0	0.9	1.7	6.6

*For those aged 45–64 years; **for those aged 75 and over.

Sources: Royal College of General Practitioners, the Office of Population Censuses and Surveys and the Department of Health *Morbidity Statistics from General Practice, Fourth National Study 1991–1992.* HMSO: London, 1995.

Mair FS, Crowley T, Bundred P. Prevalence, aetiology and management of heart failure in general practice. *Br J Gen Pract* 1996; **46**: 77–9.

Office for National Statistics (2000) *Key Health Statistics from General Practice.* The Stationery Office: London.

Davies MK, Hobbs FDR, Davis RC, *et al.* Prevalence of left-ventricular systolic dysfunction and heart failure in the Echocardiographic Heart of England Screening study: a population based study. *Lancet* 2001; **358**: 439–44.

Other sources of prevalence data: Parameshwar J, Shackell MM, Richardson A, Poole-Wilson PA, Sutton GC (1992) Prevalence of heart failure in three general practices in north west London. *Br J Gen Pract* 1992; **42**: 287–9.

Socioeconomic approach

We are accustomed to thinking of ischaemic heart disease, and by extrapolation heart failure, as strongly influenced by social class. In fact, this is not the case: the variance from the average is less than 10% for both coronary disease[38] and for heart failure in primary care.[39]

However, a major study of hospital admissions in Leicestershire gives a strikingly different picture, with four times as many first admissions for heart failure in the lowest social group as in the highest.[40] Contrasting this with the slightly lower rate of GP consultation in the lowest social class of Scottish patients, we can come up with a number of hypotheses, for example that such patients seek help late and therefore end up being admitted more frequently; but in the end the conflicting nature of the available data means that we cannot make any confident predictions about service use on the basis of social class.

Multidisciplinary care for heart failure – the unmet need

'I'm just a blood leech and monitor.' GP of Mr T

Heart failure is a complex syndrome, and many non-specialist doctors feel uneasy about dealing with it, especially in the advanced stages. Nevertheless, the vast majority of heart failure is dealt with by non-specialists – general practitioners, junior hospital doctors and consultants in medical specialties other than cardiology. Even among cardiologists, there are many whose special interests do not extend to the management of end-stage disease. This is a strikingly different situation from cancer care, where every patient is likely to receive prompt care from a range of specialists. A palliative care professional who becomes involved in the management of a cancer patient can usually be certain that the diagnosis has been clearly established and that every curative or life-prolonging intervention has been tried or at least considered. Unfortunately, this cannot yet be claimed for heart failure. The range of potential interventions for advanced heart failure is huge, yet most patients suffering from this lethal condition do not even receive an expert assessment. Small wonder that palliative care professionals, whose expertise does not include advanced cardiology, were for a long time unwilling to get involved.

Fortunately this situation is changing, albeit slowly. In the UK, the National Service Framework for Cardiovascular Disease in 2000[41] laid down a basic set of requirements for the care of heart failure, including the involvement of palliative care, and a timetable for progress. Unfortunately, in a health system which is constantly struggling with resource allocation, its targets have not been met in most localities. The basic management of heart failure was further set out in a NICE guideline for England and Wales in 2003,[42] and the need for palliative care was restated in a Department of Health guidance on service development in the same year.[43]

A great step forward has come with the deployment of heart failure nurse specialists throughout the UK over the past few years. Gradually we are seeing the coming together of the necessary elements of a heart failure team in many parts of the country (Table 1.6).

Team care is discussed in more detail in the final chapter in this book. There is no standard model, rather a number of different service configurations in widely

Table 1.6 The heart failure team

Level of care	Team members	Sources of advice/education
Day-to-day care	General practitioner Practice nurse District nurse	Primary care training courses and study days Written and online materials Advice from heart failure specialist nurse, cardiologist
Regular back-up care	Heart failure specialist nurse, community palliative care nurse, social services, heart failure clinic (community or hospital based), cardiac rehabilitation, community pharmacist Occupational therapist Physiotherapist	Accredited courses for heart failure Written and online materials Specialist courses and conferences
Specialist services	Cardiologist Geriatrician Palliative care physician Chaplain Clinical psychologist	Written materials, online materials, specialist journals Specialist courses and conferences Tertiary referral, e.g. to cardiac surgeon, interventional cardiologist

scattered locations, each resulting from local initiatives. The unmet need is still great, both for deployment of care and for the sharing of best practice between the wide range of professionals involved.

The role of palliative care services

We have seen that the palliative care needs of heart failure patients are often much wider than purely medical, and that if we are to meet them, a team approach is needed. In this context, what is the appropriate role of specialist palliative care (SPC) services, and to what extent are they willing and able to be involved?

The barriers of attitude explored by Hanratty and colleagues in their focus group study[20] a few years ago are coming down rapidly. A survey of adult SPC services in England undertaken by Louise Gibbs late in 2004[44] had a 60% response rate, with only three out of 222 respondents saying that they did not think SPCs had a role to play in end-stage heart failure. Around 60% of SPCs were already offering inpatient, day hospice and home care to such patients, albeit in small numbers only. Most SPCs expressed worries about the resource implications of taking on heart failure, but only 42% cited limited bed availability.

The educational and liaison roles of SPC are also of key importance in applying best palliative care practice to the problems of advanced heart failure. Here again the survey was encouraging, with 75% of services providing inpatient hospital support and 47% involved in outpatient hospital review. The role of the SPC services is discussed more extensively in the final chapter.

Summary

In this chapter we have seen overwhelming evidence of great need, repeatedly demonstrated over decades, but still mostly unmet. The complex syndrome of advanced heart failure, with its many accompanying physical, social, psychological and spiritual problems, presents a challenge to all professionals involved with such patients, not just those in specialist palliative care.

Because heart failure describes a wide spectrum rather than a tightly defined entity, there are few useful data to which we can turn when we attempt to estimate the likely workload for palliative care. At the same time, there is encouraging evidence that most specialist palliative care services in the UK are now willing to accept heart failure patients. In most cases this only forms a small percentage of their overall workload, but even where a more integrated service has grown up between cardiology and palliative care, this has not led to the overwhelming demand which many once feared. However, there is no established model to guide best practice, and resource restraints are widespread.

Palliative care for heart failure is now on the map, but much of the detail of the map has yet to be drawn. As we go to press, several studies of palliative care need are in different stages of completion. Merryn Gott in Sheffield and colleagues from Bradford and Exeter are near to completing an extensive survey of the palliative care needs of older people with heart failure and their families. The National Council for Palliative Care (which covers the UK except Scotland) has a cardiorespiratory working group which has undertaken a survey of existing liaison between heart failure specialist nurses and palliative care services,[45] and is planning further work. In Scotland, a study by Scott Murray and colleagues is looking at a wide range of different service models. In the near future, the need for palliative care for heart failure will be much better defined, but the more important objective is to ensure that it is met.

References

1 Hinton JM. The physical and mental distress of the dying. *QJM* 1963; **32**: 1–21.
2 Buetow S, Goodyear-Smith F, Coster G. Coping strategies in the self-management of chronic heart failure. *Fam Pract* 2001; **18**: 117–22.
3 Buetow SA, Coster G. Do general practice patients with heart failure understand its nature and seriousness, and want improved information? *Patient Educ Couns* 2001; **45**: 181–5.
4 Rogers A, Addington-Hall JM, McCoy AS *et al.* A qualitative study of chronic heart failure patients' understanding of their symptoms and drug therapy. *Eur J Heart Fail* 2002; **4**: 283–7.
5 Murray SA, Boyd K, Kendall M, Worth A, Benton TF, Clausen H. Dying of lung cancer or cardiac failure: prospective qualitative interview study of patients and their carers in the community. *BMJ* 2002; **235**: 929–34.
6 Anderson H, Ward C, Eardley A *et al.* The concerns of patients under palliative care and a heart failure clinic are not being met. *Palliat Med* 2001; **15**: 279–86.
7 Levenson JW, McCarthy EP, Lynn J, Davis RB, Phillips RS. The last six months of life for patients with congestive heart failure. *J Am Geriatr Soc* 2000; **48**(5 suppl): S101–9.
8 Nordgren L, Sorensen S. Symptoms experienced in the last six months of life with end-stage heart failure. *Eur J Cardiovasc Nurs* 2003; **2**: 213–17.
9 Hobbs FD, Kenkre JE, Roalfe AK *et al.* A cross-sectional study comparing common chronic

cardiac and medical disorders and a representative adult population. *Eur Heart J* 2002; **23**: 1867–76.

10   Murray SA, Kendall M, Boyd K, Sheikh A. Illness trajectories in palliative care. *BMJ* 2005; **330**: 1007–11.

11   Field D, Addington-Hall J. Extending specialist palliative care services to all? *Soc Sci Med* 1999; **48**: 1271–80.

12   Lunney JR, Lynn J, Foley DJ, Lipson S, Guralnik JM. Patterns of functional decline at the end of life. *JAMA* 2003; **289**: 2387–92.

13   McKinley RK, Stokes T, Exley C, Field D. Care of people dying with malignant and cardio-respiratory disease in general practice. *Br J Gen Pract* 2004; 54: 909–13.

14   Walke L, Gallo WT, Tinetti ME, Fried TR. The burden of symptoms among community-dwelling older persons with chronic advanced disease. *Arch Intern Med* 2004; **164**: 2321–4.

15   Stewart S, MacIntyre K, Hole DJ, Capewell S, McMurray JJ. More 'malignant' than cancer? Five-year survival following a first admission with heart failure. *Eur J Heart Fail* 2001; **3**: 315–22.

16   Cowie MR, Wood DA, Coats AJ *et al*. Survival of patients with a new diagnosis of heart failure: a population based study. *Heart* 2000; **83**: 505–10.

17   Murray S, Boyd K, Sheikh A. Palliative care in chronic illness [editorial]. *BMJ* 2005; **330**: 611–12.

18   Krum H, Gilbert RE. Demographics and concomitant disorders in heart failure. *Lancet* 2003; **362**: 147–58.

19   Braunstein JB, Anderson GF, Gerstenblith G *et al*. Noncardiac comorbidity increases preventable hospitalizations and mortality om Medicare beneficiaries with chronic heart failure. *J Am Coll Cardiol* 2003; **42**: 1226–33.

20   Hanratty B, Hibbert D, Mair F *et al*. Doctors' perception of palliative care for heart failure: focus group study. *BMJ* 2002; **325**: 581–5.

21   Gannon C. Palliative care in terminal cardiac failure; hospices cannot fulfil such a vast and diverse role. [letter]. *BMJ* 1995; **310**: 310–11.

22   Beattie JM, Murray RG, Brittle J, Catanheira T. Palliative care in terminal cardiac failure. Small numbers of patients with terminal cardiac failure may make considerable demands on services. [letter; comment]. *BMJ* 1995; **310**: 1411.

23   Bleumink GS, Knetsch A, Sturkenboom MC, Straus S *et al*. Quantifying the heart failure epidemic: prevalence, incidence rate, lifetime risk and prognosis of heart failure. *Eur Heart J* 2004; **18**: 1614–19.

24   Tebbit P. *Population-Based Needs Assessment for Palliative Care: a manual for cancer networks.* National Council for Palliative Care, The Cancer Action Team, London, 2004.

25   British Heart Foundation Statistics website: www.heartstats.org

26   Unal B, Critchley JA, Capewell S. Missing, mediocre, or merely obsolete? An evaluation of UK data sources for coronary heart disease. *J Epidemiol Community Health* 2003; **57**: 530–5.

27   Goldacre MJ, Mant D, Duncan M, Griffith M. Mortality from heart failure in an English population, 1979–2003: study from death certification. *J Epidemiol Community Health* 2005; **59**: 782–4.

28   AIRE data: Cleland JG, Erhardt L, Murray G, Hall AS, Ball SC. Effect of ramipril on mortality and mode of death among survivors of acute myocardial infarction with clinical evidence of heart failure. A report from the AIRE study investigators. *Eur Heart J* 1997; **18**: 41–51.

29   Poole-Wilson PA, Uretsky BF, Thygesen K, Cleland JG, Massie BM, Rydén L. Mode of death in heart failure: findings from the ATLAS trial. *Heart* 2003; **89**: 42–8.

30   British Heart Foundation Statistics website: www.heartstats.org

31   Sosin MD, Bhatia GS, Davis RC, Lip GY. Heart failure – the importance of ethnicity. *Eur J Heart Fail* 2004; **6** :831–43.

32   Joint Health Surveys Unit [2001] Health Survey for England. *The Health of Minority Ethnic Groups 1999.* The Stationery Office, London.

33 Newton JD, Blackledge HM, Squire IB. Ethnicity and variation in prognosis for patients newly hospitalised for heart failure: a matched historical cohort study. *Heart* 2005; **91**: 1545–50.

34 Sosin MD, Bhatia GS, Zafaris J, Davis RC, Lip GY. An 8-year follow-up study of acute admissions with heart failure in a multiethnic population. *Eur J Heart Fail* 2004; **6**: 669–72.

35 Galasko GI, Senior R, Lahiri A. Ethnic differences in the prevalence and aetiology of left systolic dysfunction in the community: the Harrow heart failure watch. *Heart* 2005; **91**: 595–600.

36 Blackledge HM, Newton J, Squire IB. Prognosis for South Asian and white patients newly admitted to hospital with heart failure in the United Kingdom: historical cohort study. *BMJ* 2003; **327**: 526–30.

37 Luttik ML, Jaarsma T, Moser D *et al.* The importance and impact of social support on outcomes in patients with heart failure: an overview of the literature. *J Cardiovasc Nursing* 2005; **20**: 162–9.

38 Office for National Statistics. *Key Health Statistics from General Practice*. Office for National Statistics, London, 2000.

39 MacAlister FA, Murphy NF, Simpson CR , Stewart S *et al.* Influence of socioeconomic deprivation on the primary care burden and treatment of patients with a diagnosis of heart failure in general practice in Scotland: population based study. *BMJ* 2004; **328**: 1110–13.

40 Blackledge HM, Tomlinson J, Squire IB. Prognosis for patients newly admitted to hospital with heart failure: survival trends in 12,200 index admissions in Leicestershire 1993-2001. *Heart* 2003; **89**: 615–20.

41 Department of Health. *National Service Framework for Coronary Heart Disease – modern standards and service models.* Department of Health, London, 2000.

42 NICE. *Management of Chronic Heart Failure in Adults in Primary and Secondary Care.* National Institute for Health and Clinical Excellence, London, 2003.

43 Department of Health. *Developing Services for Heart Failure.* Department of Health, London, 2003.

44 Gibbs LM, Khatri AK, Gibbs JS. Survey of Specialist Palliative Care and Heart Failure: September 2004. *Palliative Medicine.* 2006, in press.

45 National Council for Palliative Care. *A National Survey of Heart Failure Nurses and their Involvement with Palliative Care Services.* The National Council for Palliative Care, London, 2006.

Chapter 2

The syndrome of advanced heart failure

Richard Lehman

Heart failure often begins insidiously, but its end stage is a lethal syndrome which affects every organ and system in the body. In most interventional studies of NYHA class III–IV heart failure, the majority of patients are dead within two years, almost always from heart failure. Despite all the advances in treatment of the past two decades, heart failure kills because it sets in train a number of physiological and chemical responses which combine into a downward spiral.[1] On top of this, episodes of infection, inappropriate treatment or electrical instability can lead to 'decompensation', and at all stages of heart failure there is a risk of sudden death from electrical instability or new infarction.

This chapter attempts to summarise the processes of advanced heart failure for the non-specialist reader, in order to explain why heart failure tends to get worse, and why it produces its wide range of symptoms.

Aetiology

In most Western countries, around half of heart failure is due to overt ischaemia, another 40% or so is due to stiffening linked to hypertension, diabetes and ageing, and the remaining 10% is due to valvular disease or cardiomyopathy. As we saw in Chapter 1, the epidemiology of heart failure is a vexed subject, due to differences of definition, but these need not concern us here. All these processes eventually lead to the same syndrome in the final stage.

The predominant causes of heart failure differ with age:

- 0–50: congenital heart disease, cardiomyopathy
- 50–70: infarction and ischaemia
- 70–90+: increasingly a gradual onset, intermittent syndrome due to ventricular and arterial stiffening.

The age distribution of heart failure represents a summation of these processes (Figure 2.1).

The vast majority of heart failure patients are over 65 and increasingly liable to other age-related problems.

The failing pump

The traditional model of heart failure simply looked at the heart as a pump and

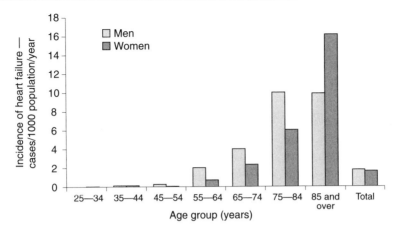

Figure 2.1 Incidence of heart failure by sex and age, 1995/96, Hillingdon. From Cowie *et al.* Incidence and aetiology of heart failure. A population-based study. *Euro Heart J* (1999); 20: 421-8. www.heartstats.org

heart failure as a mechanical process due to impaired pumping. The key factors were seen as:

- strength of contraction
- the amount of fluid in the circulation (preload)
- peripheral resistance (afterload).

Heart muscle cells are so designed that the more they are stretched, the harder they contract – this is known as Starling's Law. But when the limit is reached, ventricular failure ensues.

Failure of the right ventricle means that the systemic venous circulation cannot be cleared properly, so that peripheral venous pressure rises. This results in:

- peripheral oedema
- liver congestion
- a visibly raised jugular venous pulse (JVP).

Failure of the left ventricle means that the venous circulation of the lungs cannot be cleared properly, so that the pulmonary venous pressure rises. This results in:

- breathlessness
- orthopnoea (breathlessness worse on lying down)
- audible crackles at the lung bases.

This takes us a certain distance in understanding the symptoms of heart failure and the logic of its therapy. Preload was traditionally reduced by bleeding or leeches. Fluid and salt restriction are still used, and the traditional mainstay of heart failure treatment is the use of diuretics to expel sodium and water. Afterload can also be reduced by bleeding or leeches, but nowadays we use peripheral vasodilating drugs in three main classes – nitrates, calcium-channel blockers and angiotensin-converting enzyme inhibitors.

Using this model, it would also seem logical to use drugs that increase the contractile strength of heart muscle, known as inotropes. Such drugs are still widely used to relieve acute heart failure in hospital settings, but their long-term use is always associated with increases in mortality,[2] for reasons which will become clearer shortly.

This relatively simple model of heart failure is still a useful starting point, but it fails to explain many of the features of heart failure as a progressive syndrome. For this, we need to look in greater depth at what happens to the heart itself, and with greater breadth at the effects that this has on the rest of the body.

Cell death

The basis of the heart's pumping action is a collection of specialised muscle cells known collectively as the myocardium, and individually as cardiac myocytes. Their number, like the number of brain cells, is effectively fixed early in life, so that when they die, they are not replaced. In fact this is not *strictly* true for either heart or brain cells, but in both organs, unlike many others such as the liver or the skin, there is no effective repair mechanism to replace dead cells. The remaining cells need to work harder.

We have seen that myocytes are designed to beat harder the more they are stretched. This stretching process triggers a number of cellular mechanisms, which include the release of hormones (A- and B-type natriuretic peptides) to try to relieve preload, and an increase in myosin, which leads to the cells individually becoming bigger and stronger. This is called hypertrophy, and it results in an increase in thickness of the ventricular wall – not because there are more cells, but because the cells are bigger. These adaptive mechanisms are very effective in allowing myocytes to cope with a wide range of extra demands.

Myocytes can die by two mechanisms,[3] known by the Greek terms *necrosis* and *apoptosis*. Necrosis literally means 'turning into a corpse', referring to sudden, disorganised cell death. Apoptosis is a modern coinage meaning something like 'curling up', a programmed and orderly kind of cell death.

Necrosis of heart muscle is a common and often dramatic event witnessed every day in acute general hospitals. It is caused by the sudden occlusion of a coronary artery, leading to loss of blood supply to a segment of ventricle, usually the left. The tissue death that results is known as infarction, and it consists of the mass necrosis of cells deprived of oxygen and nutrients. Necrotic myocytes burst and release their cell contents, leading to electrical instability and the risk of sudden death from ventricular fibrillation. The infarcted segment of ventricle becomes mechanically unstable, leading to ventricular wall weakness or even rupture. If the patient survives, the necrotic area heals by a process of mass fibrosis, which can impair its blood supply further.

Apoptosis is the process of cells deciding that enough is enough. Many cells in the body are programmed to make this decision within days or weeks, and are duly replaced by similar cells. But cardiac myocytes are programmed to use apoptosis literally as the last resort, when they have been overstretched or undernourished for years or decades. The commonest reasons are long-standing hypertension, leading to chronic pathological hypertrophy, or diffuse ischaemia; diabetes is often associated with both these processes. The process of apotosis is orderly and does not cause the release of toxins or immediate electrical or mechanical instability. However, the lost myocytes are replaced only by fibrous tissue, meaning that the remaining myocytes have to work harder and may 'decide' on apoptosis sooner. In this way, the failing heart becomes progressively depleted of working cells.

Remodelling

Death of heart muscle, especially by necrosis, is followed by a process of reshaping the muscles of the entire ventricle in response to the changed distribution of mechanical load. This is called remodelling, and it can either be favourable or unfavourable for the future of the heart.[4] Favourable remodelling is a process of 'tightening up', so that the ventricle regains the size and shape which allow efficient pumping. Adverse remodelling is a process in which the damaged ventricle becomes progressively stretched. When the word 'remodelling' is used on its own in the heart failure literature (spelt 'remodeling' in US publications), it usually refers to adverse remodelling. This can be symmetrical, leading to a bigger, floppier ventricle, in which the myocytes are continuously overstretched and therefore likely to die off gradually by apoptosis. Even worse, it can be asymmetrical, in which there is a weak, bulging area of ventricular wall due to a large area of infarction. As well as making ventricular contraction less efficient, this stresses the adjacent muscle segments and carries an additional risk of electrical instability.

The renin–angiotensin–aldosterone system (RAAS)

This system of hormones is designed to preserve blood flow to the kidneys in the event of sudden haemorrhage, or some other cause for a drop in blood pressure or circulating volume. It is therefore designed to work rapidly to raise blood pressure and retain sodium and water. In other words, it is there to increase preload and keep it increased. Heart failure acts as a trigger to activate the RAAS because the failing heart sends less blood to the kidneys. This sets up a vicious cycle in which the RAAS increases preload and further overburdens the heart.

Angiotensinogen (inert substrate)

↓

is converted to   catalysed by **Renin**
   blocked by inhibitors (none yet licensed)

↓

Angiotensin I (weakly active vasoconstrictor)

↓

is converted to   catalysed by **ACE (angiotensin converting enzyme)**
   blocked by inhibitors (e.g. lisinopril, enalapril)

↓

Angiotensin II (active vasoconstrictor, vasopressor)

↓

causes release of   *blocked by angiotensin receptor blockers (ARBs, also*
   known as angiotensin II receptor antagonists (AIIAs)
   (e.g. losartan, valsartan))

↓

Aldosterone (causes further vasoconstriction, BP elevation, sodium and water retention)

Figure 2.2 The renin–angiotensin–aldosterone system (RAAS).

The RAAS has been the main target for therapeutic innovation in heart failure over the past 20 years, so that we can now potentially block every stage of the cascade. However, this is a therapeutic strategy with diminishing returns, and carries with it the danger of hyperkalaemia and hypotension if carried too far. Every patient with heart failure should be on some form of RAAS-blocking medication, but how much and how many kinds are issues that remain contentious (*see* Chapter 3).

Sympathetic nervous system

The sympathetic nervous system governs the rate of the heart either by adrenaline and noradrenaline released into the circulation, mainly from the adrenal glands, or by direct adrenergic innervation to the atrium. Once again, falling output from the failing heart triggers a response aimed at elevating blood pressure to maintain essential organ perfusion. In addition, adrenergic stimulation increases the rate of the heart in an attempt to increase cardiac output, at the same time as increasing afterload by shutting down peripheral arterioles.

Just as with RAAS activation, these are useful responses to sudden blood loss or other emergencies involving a temporary drop in circulation, but they are harmful to the failing heart in a number of ways. An increase in peripheral resistance (afterload) means that the heart has to work harder. An increase in heart rate means that the filling of the ventricles and the coronary arteries is less efficient.

Up to a decade ago, adrenergic *stimulant* drugs were being used in heart failure to increase cardiac output and improve symptoms. When it became clear that they actually increased progression and mortality, the opposite strategy was tried, and now cardioselective beta-adrenergic *blocking* drugs are used in all classes of heart failure with benefits at least as great as those of RAAS-blocking drugs.

Cardiac perfusion

Contracting myocytes need a good oxygen supply. Another vicious cycle can come about because the oxygen supply to the heart is partly dependent on the heart's own function. If there is pulmonary oedema, the oxygenation of the blood is impaired. If the heart is beating too fast, then the coronary arteries do not have time to fill properly during diastole. These factors are worsened by narrowing of the coronary arteries by atheroma and distortion of the coronary microvasculature by myocardial fibrosis.

The result may be that parts of the ventricle go into a state of paralysis known as hibernation. The myocytes are alive but inactive, and can be restored to full function by improving the delivery of oxygen to them. This is the rationale for attempting coronary reperfusion (by percutaneous procedures or by coronary artery bypass grafting) in heart failure.

Decompensation – when chronic becomes acute

In acute heart failure (decompensation), all the mechanisms that we have discussed come into play in a catastrophic sequence. Extra demand on the heart as a result of the factors listed below leads to sympathetic activation, which speeds the heart rate. This leads to impaired filling of the ventricles and the coronary arteries, producing a fall in cardiac output and a degree of ischaemic stress on the already compromised heart. The RAAS also comes into action, adding to the fluid load. Pulmonary oedema builds rapidly and further impairs oxygenation of the heart and the whole body. If the situation continues unchecked, the patient becomes cyanotic and intensely distressed, with oedema fluid frothing in the trachea. Remarkably, intravenous diamorphine usually produces immediate relief, and begins to reverse the process by relieving respiratory effort and sympathetic overdrive well before theL, which is given concurrently, has had time to work. High-concentration oxygen is also vital in this situation.

The common precipitants of decompensation are:

- infection
- arrhythmia
- anaemia
- inappropriate drug treatment, usually non-steroidal anti-inflammatory drugs
- new myocardial infarction, which may be silent
- inappropriate cessation of drug treatment
- metabolic disorders such as hyperthyroidism or uncontrolled diabetes.

Rhythm and synchrony

The proportion of heart failure patients with atrial fibrillation rises from less than 10% in NYHA class I to approximately 50% in NYHA class IV.[5] This arrhythmia greatly impairs the heart's ability to respond to changes in demand. The onset of atrial fibrillation in an already impaired heart may therefore lead to the cycle of decompensation just described.

While electrical instability of the atrium is undesirable, electrical instability of the ventricle is immediately life threatening. Episodes of ventricular tachycardia can lead to fatal ventricular fibrillation, and the best way to prevent this is by implanting a cardioverter device (ICD). This technology is expensive and raises difficult issues at the end of life, as discussed in Chapter 8.

As many as a third of heart failure patients also have impaired synchronisation between the two ventricles.[6] This can be corrected by a sophisticated and time-consuming pacing procedure known as cardiac resynchronisation therapy (CRT) or just biventricular pacing (*see* Chapter 3). This can improve life expectancy and quality of life, but availability in the UK is limited.

Skeletal muscle and cytokines

The degree of functional impairment in heart failure is poorly related to systolic function but closely related to skeletal muscle function.[7] This varies greatly between individuals and is a subject of much ongoing research.

Individuals with good skeletal muscle function can have minimal symptoms despite severe systolic impairment. Conversely, individuals with declining skeletal muscle function feel weak and breathless, lose muscle and become cachectic. They have a poor prognosis.[8]

The determinants of these differences may be partly genetic and partly due to the release of cytokines. Cytokines are a large group of chemicals that feature in the process of inflammation, and their levels are usually raised in heart failure. Many cytokines are known to trigger wasting of skeletal muscle and apoptosis of heart muscle.[9]

Struggling skeletal muscles stimulate respiratory effort and adrenergic output by means of ergoreflexes. In heart failure, these reflexes are exaggerated, and this may be another vicious circle leading to increased demand on the weakening heart.

Therapeutic approaches which have been tried are:

- blocking of cytokines, e.g. TNFα blockade with etanercept or infliximab. Unfortunately trials showed *increased* mortality in heart failure and TNFα-blocking drugs have now been shown to carry a danger of precipitating acute heart failure[10]
- muscle training programmes: these have been shown to have some short-term functional benefit but as yet no proven mortality benefit.[11]

Breathing

Breathlessness is a key feature of heart failure and the New York classification is based on it. Contributing factors are:

- pulmonary oedema – back pressure on the lung veins from an overloaded left atrium
- overdrive of the breathing muscles by chemoreceptors, which become oversensitive to carbon dioxide levels
- weakness of breathing muscles
- abnormal ventilatory patterns.

There are also characteristic changes in breathing patterns that are associated with heart failure:

- waking breathless in the night – 'paroxysmal nocturnal dyspnoea'
- breathlessness on lying down – 'orthopnoea'
- turning automatically to lie on the right side – 'trepopnoea'[12]
- long gaps in nocturnal breathing – 'apnoeic breathing patterns' or 'Cheyne-Stokes respiration'.

These breathing patterns also occur in other diseases, though trepopnoea is commonest in heart failure, and Cheyne-Stokes breathing *by day* is uncommon except in advanced heart failure.[13] In heart failure, these patterns are caused by a mixture of shifting pulmonary oedema and chemoreceptor overdrive.

There has been much interest in using continuous positive airway pressure as a treatment for the abnormal nocturnal breathing patterns of chronic heart failure, but evidence of benefit is mixed.[14] There is some evidence that nocturnal continuous oxygen may be beneficial.[15]

Nutrition and anaemia

Impaired appetite is common in heart failure and may be due to:

- congestion of the liver due to venous back-pressure
- oedema of the bowel, releasing 'feel-bad' toxins[16]
- depression.

Many non-obese patients with chronic heart failure may have an inadequate intake of calories and protein.[17] A good diet may be important in the avoidance of skeletal muscle loss and cachexia: this is an area of uncertainty and ongoing research.[18]

Anaemia is very common in heart failure.[19] Because it impairs oxygenation it can be a factor worsening failure and tipping a patient into decompensation. In advanced heart failure, most patients are anaemic to some extent and are resistant to treatment with iron alone. The anaemia of advanced heart failure is not completely understood, but it seems logical to link it with deteriorating renal function, and this is confirmed by a recent study, which found that half of the patients attending a chronic heart failure clinic had blunted endogenous production of erythropoietin associated with renal impairment.[20] Trials of treatment with synthetic erythropoietin analogues are promising.[21]

Disturbed sleep

Heart failure patients often sleep badly and wake unrefreshed.[22] This can be caused by:

- breathing disturbances
- nocturia, caused by diuretics and by disruption of the normal nightly pattern of ADH (arginine vasopressin) secretion
- depression.

Poor sleep often adds an additional burden of daytime tiredness to the fatigue already experienced by most heart failure patients.

Mood

There is an extensive literature on psychological factors in heart failure, which has been reviewed in 2002[23] and 2005.[24] Many patients with heart failure are depressed, especially the elderly.[25] Depression is associated with a worse prognosis, interacting in a complex physical way with the disease mechanisms of heart failure.[26] Pathophysiological causes of depression in advanced heart failure include:

- cytokine release, which depletes brain stores of tryptophan and hence serotonin[27]
- possible direct effects from bacterial endotoxins leaking through oedematous bowel[28]

- possible direct effects from neuroendocrine activation (increased free adrenaline and noradrenaline)
- possible direct effects from periods of brain hypoxia.

Heart failure can also lead to depression for psychosocial reasons because it is associated with:

- dependency
- weakness
- social isolation
- near-death episodes.

These are issues that need to be addressed in the holistic care of all heart failure patients. There may also be a place for some types of antidepressant drug treatment (*see* Chapter 6).

Cognitive difficulty

Many patients with heart failure experience difficulties in thinking, and heart failure is associated with a higher rate of cognitive decline and of brain tissue loss.[29] This may be due to:

- coexisting cerebrovascular disease
- periods of cerebral hypoxia caused by Cheyne-Stokes breathing
- the effect of cytokines
- anxiety/depression.

Cognitive impairment may affect the patient's ability to understand and communicate with carers and professionals, and to adhere to drug treatment. It places an added burden on those closest to the patient.

Summary

The syndrome of advanced heart failure is the result of complex disturbances of physiology and spares no system of the body. A patient with advanced heart failure will inevitably suffer from most symptoms on the following list:

- fatigue
- breathlessness
- ankle swelling
- disturbed sleep
- difficulty in concentration
- depression
- impaired appetite.

To the extent that these have physical causes, they form the 'doctor's agenda' in heart failure. However, the patient's agenda is considerably broader, as we have already glimpsed in Chapter 1 and will explore in more detail in Chapters 5 and 6. Most doctors, while recognising that their main role is in the relief of physical symptoms and the conditions that cause them, will also recognise the need to address the wider needs of the patient. This cannot be done without involving a team of professionals that can interact and communicate effectively.

References

1 Baig MK, Mahon N, McKenna WJ, Caforio AL, Bonow RO, Francis GS, Gheorghiade M. The pathophysiology of advanced heart failure. *Am Heart J* 1998; **135**: S216–S230.
2 Felker GM, O'Connor CM. Inotropic therapy for heart failure: an evidence-based approach. *Am Heart J* 2001; **142**: 393–401.
3 Kostin S, Pool L, Hein S, Drexler HC *et al*. Myocytes die by multiple mechanisms in failing human heart. *Circ Res* 2003; **92**: 715–24.
4 Gaballa MA, Goldman S. Ventricular remodelling in heart failure. *J Card Fail* 2002; **8**(6 Suppl): S476–S485.
5 Maisel WH, Stevenson LW. Atrial fibrillation in heart failure: epidemiology, pathophysiology, and rationale for therapy. *Am J Cardiol* 2003; **91**: 2D–8D.
6 McAlister FA, Ezekowitz JA, Wiebe N, Rowe B *et al*. Systematic review: cardiac resynchronization in patients with symptomatic heart failure. *Ann Intern Med* 2004; **141**: 381–90.
7 Clark AL. Origin of symptoms in chronic heart failure. *Heart* 2006; **92**: 12–16.
8 Anker SD, Coats AJ. Cardiac cachexia: a syndrome with impaired survival and immune and neuroendocrine activation. *Chest* 1999; **115**: 836–47.
9 Sharma R, Anker SD. Cytokines, apoptosis and cachexia: the potential for TNF antagonism. *Int J Cardiol* 2002; **85**: 161–71.
10 Anker SD, von Haehling S. Inflammatory mediators in chronic heart failure: an overview. *Heart* 2004; **90**: 464–70.
11 Smart N, Marwick TH. Exercise training for patients with heart failure: a systematic review of factors that improve mortality and morbidity. *Am J Med* 2004; **116**: 693–706.
12 Leung RS, Bowman ME, Parker JD, Newton GE, Bradley TD. Avoidance of the left lateral decubitus position during sleep in patients with heart failure: relationship to cardiac size and function. *J Am Coll Cardiol* 2003; **41**: 227–30.
13 Ferrier K, Campbell A, Yee B, Richards M *et al*. Sleep-disordered breathing occurs frequently in stable outpatients with congestive heart failure. *Chest* 2005; **128**: 2116–22.
14 Bradley TD, Logan AG, Kimoff RJ, Series F, Morrison D *et al*. Continuous positive airway pressure for central sleep apnea and heart failure. *N Engl J Med* 2005; **353**: 2025–33.
15 Sasayama S, Izumi T, Ueshima K, Asanoi H; CHF-HOT Study Group. Effects of nocturnal oxygen therapy on outcome measures in patients with chronic heart failure and Cheyne-Stokes respiration. *Circ J* 2006; **70**: 1–7.
16 Krack A, Sharma R, Figulla HR, Anker SD. The importance of the gastrointestinal system in the pathogenesis of heart failure. *Eur Heart J* 2005; **26**: 2368–74.
17 Aquilani R, Opasich C, Verri M, Boschi F, Febo O, Pasini E, Pastoris O. Is nutritional intake adequate in chronic heart failure patients? *J Am Coll Cardiol* 2003; **42**: 1218–23.
18 de Lorgeril M, Salen P, Defaye P. Importance of nutrition in chronic heart failure patients. *Eur Heart J* 2005; **26**: 2215–17.
19 Lindenfeld J. Prevalence of anemia and effects on mortality in patients with heart failure. *Am Heart J* 2005; **149**: 391–401.
20 Pasich C, Cazzola M, Scelsi L, Bosimini E *et al*. Blunted erythropoietin production and defective iron supply for erythropoiesis as major causes of anaemia in patients with chronic heart failure. *Eur Heart J* 2005; **26**: 2232–7.

21 van der Meer P, Voors A, Lipsic E, van Gilst WH, van Veldhuisen DJ. Erythropoietin in cardiovascular diseases. *Eur Heart J* 2004; **25**: 285–91.

22 Brostrom A, Johansson P. Sleep disturbances in patients with chronic heart failure and their holistic consequences. *Eur J Cardiovasc Nurs* 2005; **4**: 183–97.

23 MacMahon KM, Lip GY. Psychological factors in heart failure. *Arch Intern Med* 2002; **162**: 509–16.

24 Konstam V, Moser DK, De Jong MJ. Depression and anxiety in heart failure. *J Card Fail* 2005; **11**: 455–63.

25 Gottlieb SS, Khatta M, Friedmann E *et al.* The influence of age, gender, and race on the prevalence of depression in heart failure patients. *J Am Coll Cardiol* 2004; **43**: 1542–9.

26 Pasic J, Levy WC, Sullivan MD. Cytokines in depression and heart failure. *Psychosom Med* 2003; **65**: 181–93.

27 Fekertich AK, Ferguson JP, Binkley PF. Depressive symptoms and inflammation among heart failure patients. *Am Heart J* 2005; **150**: 132–6.

28 Genth-Zotz S, von Haehling S, Bolger AP *et al.* Pathophysiologic quantities of endo-toxin-induced tumor necrosis factor-alpha release in whole blood from patients with chronic heart failure. *Am J Cardiol* 2002; **90**: 1226–30.

29 Woo MJ, Macey PM, Keens PT, Kumar R *et al.* Functional abnormalities in brain areas that mediate autonomic nervous system control in advanced heart failure. *J Card Fail* 2005; **11**: 437–46.

Chapter 3

Maximum therapy for heart failure

Michael Davies

Standard medical therapy in the treatment of heart failure is a combination of a loop diuretic, an angiotensin-converting enzyme (ACE) inhibitor and a beta-blocker. A number of other pharmacological and non-pharmacological therapies are also available, and may be highly useful in selected patients. This chapter is written to offer a practical guide to the use of these different agents in an attempt to approach optimal and then as-required maximal medical therapy in heart failure. The chapter is structured under the headings of class of agents.

Patients with heart failure are invariably on a great deal of medication. The evidence base for treating heart failure has been built up by adding one drug class to another and looking for mortality benefit. This usually, but not always, equates with symptomatic benefit. Unfortunately, there is currently no way of individualising drug treatment, and most classes of drug are increased to the limit of patient toleration by a process of trial and error. But patients and doctors alike often find it difficult to know whether particular symptoms – tiredness, giddiness or cough, for example – are due to the condition itself or to the drugs treating it. Those looking after patients with advanced heart failure therefore have a difficult job deciding whether to add further treatment or to modify existing treatment.

Diuretics

Furosemide, bumetanide

Patients with heart failure and signs of fluid retention all require the use of diuretics, at least initially. The standard therapy is furosemide, which can usually be started as oral therapy. A reasonable starting dose is 40 mg but this may need to be increased, depending on the level of fluid retention and the response to an initial dose. The other group of patients who benefit significantly from a loop diuretic are those patients with significant symptomatic dyspnoea from fluid overload. This symptom may respond promptly to the use of a loop diuretic.

When patients have achieved stability, they can learn to adjust the dose of their loop diuretic according to changes in their weight. This depends on establishing a baseline optimal weight when the patient is stable. A useful indicator is an increase over a two-day period of 3 kg in weight or the detection by the patient of a recurrence of ankle swelling. In these instances it is reasonable to allow the patient to manage their own diuretic dose and to increase the dose of furosemide by an additional 40 mg daily until their optimal weight is regained – underscoring the need to give the patient their target weight, which can be assessed when they are free of overt heart failure. Diuretic dosage may need to be reduced in hot climates if patients travel abroad, or similarly decreased if patients develop intercurrent diarrhoea and vomiting. A number of patients can be stabilised on 40–80 mg of a loop diuretic daily. If symptoms deteriorate as the disease progresses, the dose of diuretic can be increased to furosemide 120–160 mg daily. In general, except perhaps in patients with concomitant renal disease, increasing the dosage above 160 mg daily of furosemide has little further benefit. If patients develop significant fluid retention again during the course of their disease, or develop worsening of their dyspnoea, it is possible that furosemide is not being adequately absorbed because of associated gut oedema. In these instances it is helpful to consider switching the loop diuretic to bumetanide on the basis that 1 mg of bumetanide is equivalent to 40 mg of furosemide. This may be better absorbed and result in an improvement in diuresis, and an improvement in symptomatology and a regain of their optimal weight. In patients with an acute deterioration in their heart failure, intravenous therapy may be required, and this may necessitate hospitalisation, although this is not always essential, given that some patients respond rapidly to two or three days of intravenous furosemide therapy and can then return to oral loop diuretic treatment.

As with all loop diuretics it is essential to avoid hypokalaemia and potassium supplementation or the addition of a potassium-sparing diuretic, i.e. amiloride or spironolactone (see below), may be helpful. Overdiuresis should also be remembered, and the tired patient with dizziness on standing and a corresponding postural drop in blood pressure should have their loop diuretic dose reviewed.

Spironolactone, eplerenone

Recent studies have shown that adding the anti-aldosterone agent spironolactone at low doses (25 mg daily) to a loop diuretic and an ACE inhibitor in patients with NYHA class III–IV heart failure can result in additional improvement in symptoms and a reduction in mortality. This was shown in the RALES study.[1] The EPHESUS study[2] confirmed beneficial effects from the use of eplerenone in patients with left ventricular dysfunction shortly after myocardial infarction. The aldosterone antagonist eplerenone may therefore be a useful alternative to spironolactone. It has no oestrogenic action and therefore avoids some of the troublesome side effects of spironolactone, such as gynaecomastia and nausea. An aldosterone antagonist should be added for patients who remain significantly symptomatic despite a loop diuretic and an ACE inhibitor. With both spironolactone and eplerenone, renal function on commencement of therapy needs to be carefully monitored and the dose adjusted if there is a significant rise in creatinine or potassium levels, particularly as these patients are also on an ACE inhibitor, which retains potassium. Cases of fatal hyperkalaemia have been reported following the use of aldosterone antagonists, and it is prudent to check the potassium one week and three weeks following each dose change.

Metolazone

In patients with resistant overt heart failure the addition of a thiazide-like diuretic, metolazone, may be helpful. This is usually given in a dose of 2.5–5 mg daily initially. The effect may not be seen for 2 to 4 days and then a pronounced diuresis may occur. It is important in this instance to ensure that the dose of metolazone is reduced to perhaps 2.5 mg on alternate days, and many patients, having developed a satisfactory diuresis, can be maintained on a combination of a loop diuretic and twice-weekly metolazone.

Summary points – diuretics

- Most patients require a loop diuretic and many can be managed well on furosemide.
- If patients remain significantly symptomatic despite a loop diuretic and an ACE inhibitor, the addition of spironolactone or eplerenone should be considered.
- If patients develop progressive heart failure despite optimal medical therapy, up-titration of their diuretic dose, switching to a different loop diuretic or adding in metolazone may be beneficial.
- Careful monitoring of renal function and electrolytes is important.
- Loop diuretics can be self-managed by patients who have been taught to monitor their weight.
- Overdiuresis can result in postural dizziness and fatigue and should be looked for.

Angiotensin-converting enzyme inhibitors

There is a large evidence base of interventional trials illustrating the beneficial effects of a large number of ACE inhibitors in all stages/grades of heart failure.[3-9] This includes beneficial effects on morbidity, the rate of progression of heart failure and mortality. ACE inhibitors have been shown to be beneficial in the prevention of left ventricular dilatation following myocardial infarction (coronary heart disease is the commonest cause of heart failure) and have been shown to reduce the rate of progression of asymptomatic heart failure (NYHA class I) to symptomatic heart failure (progression to NYHA class II–IV). Furthermore, ACE inhibitors have been shown to reduce morbidity and mortality in all classes of symptomatic heart failure – beneficial effects being shown in class II, class III and in severe heart failure (class IV). As mentioned above, optimal medical therapy consists of a diuretic in addition to an ACE inhibitor and then subsequently the use of beta-blockers. All patients with left ventricle (LV) dysfunction, whether symptomatic or asymptomatic, should therefore be considered for an ACE inhibitor. Initiation should be with low doses, but patients should be titrated up to the maximum tolerated dose within manufacturer's guidelines. There is evidence that although some benefit is accrued in treating patients with low-dose ACE inhibitors, further benefits are obtained using higher doses.[10] The majority of clinical trials relate to the use of doses titrated up to the maximum tolerated dose. Intuitively, it is also advisable to use long-acting ACE inhibitors rather than short-acting ACE inhibitors, as more complete 24-hour ACE inhibition may be obtained and adherence to treatment is simplified.

A variety of ACE inhibitors are available, and some of these have ancillary properties that may be beneficial, but the most important thing is to establish the patient on an ACE inhibitor, and for the majority of patients this can be done safely in primary care. It is essential that they are regularly reviewed in primary care to up-titrate doses, providing this is well tolerated clinically, haemodynamically, and in terms of their renal function and electrolyte results. Markers to suggest that first-dose hypotension may be problematic include hyponatraemia, a resting tachycardia (heart rate greater than 100), hypotension (systolic blood pressure less than 100), the use of other concomitant vasodilators (i.e. nitrates), and unstable heart failure. In patients who do not have overt fluid retention, an ACE inhibitor can be started before a loop diuretic. In patients who have significant limiting dyspnoea or overt fluid retention, a loop diuretic is helpful in the first instance, and when the patient is stabilised and free of overt fluid retention an ACE inhibitor can be commenced.

Up to 10–20% of patients cannot tolerate an ACE inhibitor because of side effects. Sometimes these are dose related, and so adjustment to lower doses may be useful. The commonest side effect is cough, due to impaired bradykinin clearance from the upper airway, and this is a class effect of all ACE inhibitors. A useful alternative is an angiotensin II receptor blocking agent. The effectiveness of an angiotensin II receptor blocking agent has recently been underscored in the CHARM[11] study, using candesartan in patients with chronic heart failure, and in the VALIANT study[12] (using valsartan) in patients following myocardial infarction. There is also evidence to support the use of an angiotensin II receptor blocking agent as an alternative agent to an ACE inhibitor in patients who are not able to tolerate an ACE inhibitor in the Val-HeFT study, using valsartan.[13] Again, low doses should be prescribed initially as with ACE inhibitors and the dose titrated upwards to the maximum tolerated dose within the manufacturer's guidelines. One of the study arms in the CHARM results related to the additive effects of candesartan to an ACE inhibitor.[14] Beneficial effects were gained, and it may be that in the future, this is a further useful therapeutic approach to patients with significant heart failure despite adequate treatment with a loop diuretic and an ACE inhibitor with or without a beta-blocker. In the case of candesartan, there was no compromised effect in patients where additional beta blockade was used, i.e. in patients on triple therapy consisting of an ACE inhibitor, a beta-blocker and additional candesartan.

In patients where neither an ACE inhibitor nor an angiotensin II receptor blocking agent can be tolerated, alternative vasodilatation can be achieved with a combination of hydralazine and an isosorbide nitrate, as used in some of the early trials in heart failure. Isosorbide preparations may also be useful agents in patients where the underlying aetiology for the heart failure is ischaemic heart disease.

If a patient's creatinine rises significantly with the use of an ACE inhibitor, it is not always necessary to down-titrate this agent – an alternative is to look to see if a reduction in loop diuretic dosage can be achieved, which may result in an improvement in creatinine. If the creatinine does not respond to a reduction in diuretic dosage then the ACE inhibitor may need to be down-titrated, but perhaps with some loss of beneficial long-term effects.

Summary points – ACE inhibitors

- There is strong evidence showing that ACE inhibitors help prevent the development of heart failure, and in those with heart failure, to slow progression of disease, improve symptoms and improve survival.
- Initiation should be low doses, and titrated upwards.
- 'First-dose hypotension' is more common if there is hyponatraemia, tachycardia, hypotension, use of other vasodilators, unstable heart failure or high-dose loop diuretics.
- Once stabilised, the dose of loop diuretic required may be less.
- If the serum creatinine rises despite a reduction in loop diuretic, then the ACE inhibitor may need to be down-titrated.
- 10–20% of patients cannot tolerate an ACE inhibitor because of cough. In these patients, an angiotensin II receptor blocker may be a useful alternative.

Patients with symptomatic heart failure due to left ventricular systolic dysfunction should be treated with the following drugs (if tolerated and not contraindicated) and in the sequence indicated. The reader must refer to the text of the guideline (*see* www.nice.org.uk) for more detailed discussion and explanation.

Please note:
- Diuretic is first-line therapy when a patient presents with acute pulmonary oedema.
- Please refer to Appendix D of NICE guideline for starting doses of drugs.
- The arrow on the left-hand margin indicates the increasing likelihood of the need for specialist input.

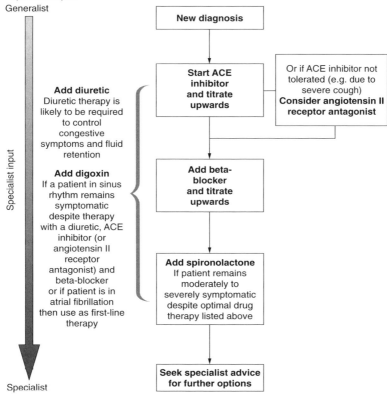

Figure 3.1 Algorithm for the pharmacological treatment of symptomatic heart failure due to left ventricular systolic dysfunction. *See* www.nice.org.uk

Beta-adrenergic blocking agents

Substantial beneficial effects may be seen in terms of morbidity and mortality with the addition of a beta-blocker for patients with heart failure on a loop diuretic and an ACE inhibitor.[15–17] This has been repeatedly shown in a number of different studies involving a variety of beta-blocking agents – in particular carvedilol, bisoprolol and metoprolol. It is now routine practice to establish patients on an ACE inhibitor and loop diuretic and then to initiate beta-blocker therapy. Again, very low doses should be used, and the dose interval between titration should be a minimum of two weeks. At the present time, the majority of patients can be established on diuretics and ACE inhibitors in primary care but then require referral to specialist heart failure services (nurse and/or medical practitioner-led services) for the initiation and up-titration of beta-blocker therapy. There is always the potential risk of decompensation on starting a beta-blocker in heart failure, but this is surprisingly low providing the patient is stable and the recommendations of low doses and slow up-titration are followed. Parameters monitored for the determination of up-titration of a beta-blocker include changes in symptoms (particularly an increase in dyspnoea, suggesting an even slower up-titration), daily weight, systolic blood pressure and pulse rate. The usual contraindications relating to asthma apply.

Summary points – beta-blockers

- There is strong evidence that the addition of a beta-blocker improves both morbidity and mortality.
- It is now routine practice to establish the patient on a loop diuretic and ACE inhibitor, then add in a beta-blocker.
- Up-titration must be done slowly.
- There is a risk of decompensation, but this appears to be small if the patient was stable at initiation.
- Beta-blockers are contraindicated in patients with asthma.

Aims of therapy

The main aims of therapy are to improve symptoms and quality of life, and reduce hospital admissions (all are measures of improved morbidity), as well as improving mortality. Although no randomised controlled trial of loop diuretics has demonstrated improved mortality, this is undoubtedly the case, and therefore all the above classes of compound achieve these aims. In addition, ACE inhibitors and beta-blockers may slow the progression of deterioration of heart failure. For these reasons the aim should be to establish all patients on an ACE inhibitor and beta-blocker. It is always important to remember that it may be possible to reduce the dose of a loop diuretic once the patient is established on adequate doses of ACE inhibition and beta-blocker therapy.

Digoxin

Atrial fibrillation may be the cause of heart failure in a number of patients, i.e. the patients may present with all the symptoms and some of the signs of heart failure, but their LV systolic function may be relatively well maintained or even normal, and the primary abnormality is uncontrolled atrial fibrillation. In addition, up to 30% of patients with significant LV dysfunction have concomitant atrial fibrillation. Digoxin obviously has an important role to play in both these patient groups. In these instances, control of heart rate may result in significant symptomatic improvement. In addition, some patients with otherwise chronic stable heart failure may deteriorate because of the development of atrial fibrillation. If significant improvement is not obtained with rate control with the use of digoxin, these patients may be candidates for consideration for cardioversion. However, success rates may be low if there is an underlying cardiac structural abnormality, i.e. left ventricular and/or left atrial dilatation. The beneficial effects of digoxin in these groups of patients are primarily due to the electrophysiological effects of digoxin slowing atrioventricular (AV) nodal conduction.

Some patients with heart failure due to LV systolic dysfunction may benefit from digoxin even if in sinus rhythm. This may be partly due to the weak inotropic (strengthened contraction of the heart cells) effect of digoxin. The beneficial inotropic effects of digoxin have been sought in a number of trials over many years, and meta-analyses have shown that a few patients may benefit. It is therefore worth considering digoxin in patients who have ongoing symptomatic heart failure in sinus rhythm despite the use of loop diuretics, ACE inhibitors, beta-blockers and aldosterone antagonists (spironolactone or eplerenone). As ever with the use of digoxin, normokalaemia should be maintained as both hypo- and hyperkalaemia may result in significant deleterious effects of digoxin increasing the risk of arrhythmias.

Anticoagulant therapy

All patients with heart failure and atrial fibrillation should be considered for concomitant warfarin therapy, and warfarin used unless it is significantly contraindicated. The risk of thromboembolism is high in patients with dilated poorly functioning ventricles and heart failure, and also the left atrium is often dilated. The question of anticoagulation in sinus rhythm is more difficult to answer.[18] However, if on echocardiography there is evidence of left ventricular or left atrial clot, then warfarin is certainly indicated.

Aspirin

The commonest cause for heart failure is coronary heart disease. Aspirin is routinely used in patients following myocardial infarction and in patients with angina. This is due to the beneficial effects on primary and secondary prevention in terms of coronary thrombosis, and aspirin should be maintained in patients with heart failure where the underlying aetiology is coronary artery disease. There is a question of aspirin offsetting some of the beneficial effects of ACE inhibitors through bradykinin pathways, but the beneficial effects in terms of coronary artery disease probably offset any effect on reducing the efficacy of ACE inhibitors.

Natural history of heart failure

All grades of heart failure carry a poor prognosis. The natural history of heart failure is usually one of progressive disease despite optimal medical therapy, or the occurrence of sudden death. The decline may occur slowly over time or rapidly. In addition, the patient may continue with stable symptoms for some time, punctuated by episodes of acute decompensation often requiring hospitalisation. Following adjustment of their medical therapy, patients may return to their previous level of symptoms or improve significantly but retain a level of further symptomatic impairment. In patients on optimal therapy, a number of well-recognised causes of decompensation are listed in Table 3.1.

Acute decompensation

Once heart failure treatment is stabilised, it is important to prevent decompensation whenever possible. Intercurrent chest infections can be reduced by routine immunisation against influenza and pneumococcal infections. Patient compliance always needs checking: the better the patient understands the purpose of drug treatment, the less likely that poor compliance will play a significant role in decompensation. This is also true in relation to attention to daily salt and fluid intake. As mentioned above, atrial fibrillation may be a significant cause for acute decompensation in a previously stable heart failure patient.

Further intercurrent events, particularly further myocardial infarction or further acute ischaemic episodes, may result in significant deterioration (albeit only transiently in some) in LV function. Ischaemic heart disease is the commonest cause of heart failure and therefore intercurrent ischaemic events may play an important role in decompensation/deterioration in a significant number of patients. Beta-adrenergic receptor blocking agents and isosorbide preparations are useful agents in patients where the underlying aetiology for the heart failure is ischaemic heart disease, providing treatment for both the heart failure and the underlying ischaemic aetiology. In this group of patients, calcium antagonists may cause problems due to negative inotropic effects and probably the agent of

Table 3.1 Causes of acute decompensation

- Infection
- Arrhythmia
- Anaemia
- Inappropriate drug treatment, usually non-steroidal anti-inflammatory drugs
- New myocardial infarction, which may be silent
- Inappropriate cessation of drug treatment
- Metabolic disorders such as hyperthyroidism or uncontrolled diabetes

---

choice in this group of compounds would be amlodipine. It is worth remembering that exercise testing, radionuclide imaging and coronary angiography should be considered in heart failure patients to determine first, the correct underlying aetiology, and second, whether revascularisation would be helpful to improve cardiac function and/or prevent further myocardial loss.

Decompensation may result from other arrhythmias such as ventricular tachycardia, or pulmonary emboli or other intercurrent infections causing fever and vasodilatation. It is important to try to establish the cause of acute decompensation as this may allow targeted therapy to the primary decompensating cause.

Many patients with decompensated heart failure will require hospital admission. This, however, may not always be the case and depends very much on the severity of the decompensation and how acute this is. If it is a gradual process, then adjustment to diuretic dose and type with the addition of other diuretics as mentioned above may restabilise their heart failure. If patients develop severe and acute decompensation, admission is usually required. Up to 5% of all medical admissions are for heart failure and therefore this is an important and widespread problem in terms of patient care and the use of resources. Many of the guidelines relating to heart failure have focused on chronic heart failure, but the European Society of Cardiology has issued guidelines on the management of acute heart failure.[19]

The National Service Framework for coronary heart disease has promoted the establishment of diagnostic and treatment services for heart failure patients. This has resulted over the past few years in dedicated open-access heart failure clinics and the establishment of an increasingly widespread heart failure specialist nurse service. Lead consultants in heart failure are identified in many trusts. Patients with acute decompensated heart failure are usually admitted via the acute medical take, but it is always beneficial to consider, dependent on local circumstances, whether liaison with the heart failure specialist nurses and/or lead consultant in heart failure may avoid hospitalisation or perhaps allow admission under the most appropriate specialty. The fact is that heart failure is managed in primary care for the majority of patients and for the majority of time, but at times of acute decompensation hospital care may be required. This underscores the importance of liaison pathways for these patients between primary and secondary/tertiary care. In some areas, heart failure specialist nurses work between primary care and the local hospital trust and therefore the possibilities of very close liaison are enhanced.

Acute decompensation in previously diagnosed and treated chronic heart failure patients (as opposed to acute heart failure *de novo*) may be difficult to treat. There is a reliance on the use of intravenous diuretics and supplemental oxygen therapy as well as short-term intravenous inotropic support. There is no real consensus on the relative usefulness of the various intravenous inotropes, but the most frequent practice is to commence patients on intravenous dobutamine/dopamine. Other inotropes (and other pharmacological agents) may be added to or used instead of intravenous dobutamine. These include adrenaline, noradrenaline and phosphodiesterase inhibitors, i.e. enoximone. Inotropes may be used in one of a number of ways – as a bridge to recovery, as a bridge to establishment on further medical or non-pharmacological (including device) therapy, or as a bridge to transplantation – dependent on the situation and appropriateness for the individual patient. In many patients, short-term intravenous diuretic and inotropic therapy may result in a return to their previous level of symptom control. In other patients, inotropic support may allow the introduction of further medical therapy, i.e. increased doses of ACE inhibitors or the addition of metolazone or other agents, and again achieve a significant degree of symptom relief. In younger patients with acute decompensation despite optimal therapy, cardiac transplantation may be an option, either during an episode of acute decompensation or following such an episode successfully treated with intravenous therapy.

Device therapy

Various non-pharmacological options are available to both patients with chronic stable heart failure and patients with acute decompensated heart failure.

Biventricular pacing

Cardiac resynchronisation therapy (CRT) may result in substantial improvement in some patients who remain significantly limited by dyspnoea despite optimal medical therapy.[20] Although it may be difficult to predict which patients will improve significantly, biventricular pacing should be considered in patients who remain significantly symptomatic on optimal medical treatment and who have a broad QRS complex and a significantly impaired ejection fraction. Obviously this may be appropriate only in selected patients, but substantial improvements may be seen in some patients – overall, approximately 70% of patients may show a positive response to treatment.

Implantable defibrillators

Again, careful patient selection is important, but implantable defibrillators improve mortality in patients with significantly impaired LV function and high-grade ventricular arrhythmias.[21] The current NICE guidelines for considering patients for implantable defibrillators are given in Table 3.2.

Modern technology now also provides for combined CRT and implantable defibrillators, and recent studies address the relative merits of these.

Left ventricular assist devices

Even more selective groups of patients may need to be considered for these devices and again the benefits can be subdivided into a bridge to recovery, a bridge to transplantation or as a permanent therapy. A number of left ventricular assist devices (LVADs) are available, but the results of large trials are awaited. Undoubtedly these may allow all three objectives to be achieved, but particularly at present in the first two areas as a bridge to recovery and as a bridge to transplantation. Again, it depends very much on the suitability of the patient, particularly in relation to co-morbid diseases and ultimate prognosis.

Table 3.2 Implantable cardioverter defibrillators for arrhythmias: NICE guidance January 2006

This appraisal does not cover the use of implantable defibrillators for non-ischaemic dilated cardiomyopathy

1.1   ICDs are recommended for patients in the following categories.

1.1.1 Secondary prevention,* that is, for patients who present, in the absence of a treatable cause, with one of the following:
  • having survived a cardiac arrest due to either ventricular tachycardia (VT) or ventricular fibrillation (VF)
  • spontaneous sustained VT causing syncope or significant haemodynamic compromise
  • sustained VT without syncope or cardiac arrest, and who have an associated reduction in ejection fraction (LVEF of less than 35%) (no worse than class III of the New York Heart Association functional classification of heart failure).

1.1.2 Primary prevention,† that is, for patients who have:
  • a history of previous (more than 4 weeks) myocardial infarction (MI) and:

either
– left ventricular dysfunction with an LVEF of less than 35% (no worse than class III of the New York Heart Association functional classification of heart failure)

and
– non-sustained VT on holter (24-hour electrocardiogram [ECG]) monitoring

and
– inducible VT on electrophysio-logical (EP) testing

or
– left ventricular dysfunction with an LVEF of less than 30% (no worse than class III of the New York Heart Association functional classification of heart failure)

and
– QRS duration of equal to or more than 120 milliseconds

  • a familial cardiac condition with a high risk of sudden death, including long QT syndrome, hypertrophic cardiomyopathy, Brugada   syndrome   or arrhythmogenic right ventricular dysplasia, or have undergone surgical repair of congenital heart disease

---

* Secondary prevention of sudden cardiac death (SCD) is defined as the prevention of an additional life-threatening event in survivors of sudden cardiac events or in patients with recurrent unstable rhythms.

† Primary prevention of SCD is defined as prevention of a first life-threatening arrhythmic event.

Cardiac transplantation

Carefully selected patients may be candidates for cardiac transplantation. Younger patients with end-stage heart failure are obvious candidates and cardiac transplantation may frequently lead to considerable improvement in morbidity and considerable improvements in prognosis at least in the short to medium term.

Organisation of services

As mentioned previously, the National Service Framework for coronary heart disease has enhanced the services and facilities for patients with suspected and confirmed heart failure. Open-access diagnostic clinics are improving the quality of diagnosis, and optimal management is dependent on accurate diagnosis. In addition open-access heart failure clinics allow for improvements in pharmaco-logical therapy and patient education. Routine up-titration of ACE inhibitor therapy and then routine establishment and up-titration of beta-blocker therapy is enhanced. A key development has been the training and deployment of heart failure specialist nurses. Specialist nurses can improve patient understanding and adherence to treatment, monitor and advise on day-to-day problems, and report on the patient's progress. Where available, they are important links in communication between primary care, local hospital services and palliative care. The establishment of consultants and general practitioners with specialist inter-est in heart failure also improves the treatment and follow-up of patients with this disease, which is associated with a generally poor prognosis. The majority of patients are managed in primary care for most of the time, and primary care nurses can be an invaluable help in the day-to-day management and monitoring of heart failure treatment. The hospital setting becomes important when patients fail to respond adequately to medical therapy, develop episodes of acute decom-pensation or require more specialist intervention, including device therapy and cardiac transplantation.

Palliative care

Patients with heart failure are somewhat different from those usually referred for palliative care. They can oscillate between being relatively well controlled, even though with quite limiting symptoms, to having severe life-threatening heart failure. The involvement of palliative care services for these patients may there-fore be intermittent, and substantial improvements (at least temporary) may punctuate the gradual progressive nature of the condition. One of the worst symptoms of any disease is dyspnoea, and in heart failure there are many thera-pies that may improve this, even in the end stages of the condition. These include the use of intravenous diuretics and opioids together with supplemental oxygen therapy, as discussed further in Chapter 5. Intravenous or transdermal nitrates may also improve dyspnoea in some patients and should always be considered in patients with terminal heart failure. These may produce a fall in cardiac pressures sufficient to reduce pulmonary congestion.

References

1 Pitt B, Zannad F, Remme WJ *et al*. The effect of spironolactone on morbidity and mortality in patients with severe heart failure. *N Eng J Med* 1999: **341**: 709–17.
2 Pitt B, Remme WJ, Zannad F *et al*. Eplerenone, a selective aldosterone blocker, in

patients with left ventricular dysfunction after myocardial infarction. *N Eng J Med* 2003: **348**: 1309–21.

3   The SOLVD Investigators. Effect of enalapril on mortality and the development of heart failure in asymptomatic patients with reduced ejection fractions. *N Eng J Med* 1992: **327**: 685–91.

4   The SOLVD Investigators. Effect of enalapril on survival in patients with reduced left ventricular ejection fractions and congestive heart failure. *N Eng J Med* 1991: **325**: 293–302.

5   Cohn JN, Johnson MS, Ziesche S *et al*. A comparison of enalapril with hydralazine-isosorbide dinitrate in the treatment of chronic congestive cardiac failure. *N Eng J Med* 1991: **325**: 303–10.

6   The CONSENSUS Trial Study Group. Effects of enalapril on mortality in severe heart failure. *N Eng J Med* 1987: **316**: 1429–35.

7   Pfeffer MA, Braunwald E, Moye LA *et al*. Effect of captopril on mortality and morbidity in patients with left ventricular dysfunction after myocardial infarction. *N Eng J Med* 1992: **327**: 669–77.

8   Kober L, Torp-Pedersen C, Carlsen JE *et al*. A clinical trial of the angiotensin-converting-enzyme inhibitor trandolapril in patients with left ventricular dysfunction after myocardial infarction. *N Eng J Med* 1995: **333**: 1670–6.

9   The Acute Infarction Ramipril Efficiency (AIRE) Study Investigators. Effect of ramipril on mortality and morbidity of survivors of acute myocardial infarction with clinical evidence of heart failure. *Lancet* 1993; **342**: 821–8.

10 Packer M, Poole-Wilson PA, Armstrong PW *et al*. Comparative effects of low dose and high doses of the angiotensin converting enzyme inhibitor, lisinopril, on morbidity and mortality in chronic heart failure. *Circulation* 1999; **100**: 2312–18.

11 Granger CB, McMurray JJV, Yusuf S *et al*. Effects of candesartan in patients with chronic heart failure and reduced left ventricular systolic function intolerant to angiotensin-converting-enzyme inhibitors: the CHARM-Alternative trial. *Lancet* 2003; **362**: 772–6.

12 Pfeffer MA, McMurray JJV, Velazquez EJ *et al*. Valsartan, captopril, or both in myocardial infarction complicated by heart failure, left ventricular dysfunction, or both. *N Eng J Med* 2003: **349**: 1893–906.

13 Cohn JN, Tognoni G for the Valsartan Heart Failure Trial Investigators. A randomised trial of the angiotensin-receptor blocker valsartan in chronic heart failure. *N Eng J Med* 2001; **345**: 1667–75.

14 McMurray JJV, Ostergen J, Swedberg K *et al*. Effects of candesartan in patients with chronic heart failure and reduced left ventricular systolic function taking angiotensin-converting-enzyme inhibitors: the CHARM-Added trial. *Lancet* 2003; **362**: 761–71,

15 CIBIS II Investigators. The cardiac insufficiency bisoprolol study II (CIBIS II): a randomised trial. *Lancet* 1999; **353**: 9–13.

16 Packer M, Bristow MR, Cohn JN *et al*. The effect of carvedilol on morbidity and mortality in patients with chronic heart failure. *N Eng J Med* 1996; **334**: 1349–55.

17 MERIT-HF Study Group. Effect of metoprolol CR/XL in chronic heart failure: Metoprolol CR/XL randomised intervention trial in congestive heart failure (MERIT-HF). *Lancet* 1999; **353**: 2001–9.

18 Cleland JG, Findlay I, Jafri S *et al*. The Warfarin/Aspirin Study in Heart failure (WASH): a randomised trial comparing antithrombotic strategies for patients with heart failure. *Am Heart J* 2004; **148**: 157–64.

19 Nieminen MS, Bohm M, Cowie MR *et al*. Executive summary of the guidelines on the diagnosis and treatment of acute heart failure: the Task Force on Acute Heart Failure of the European Society of Cardiology. *Eur Heart J* 2005; **26**: 384–416.

20 Cleland JF, Daubert JC, Erdmann E *et al*. The effect of cardiac resynchronisation on morbidity and mortality in heart failure. *N Eng J Med* 2005; **352**: 1539–49.

21 Moss AJ, Hall WJ, Cannon DS *et al*. Improved survival with an implanted defibrillator in patients with coronary disease at high risk for ventricular arrhythmia. *N Eng J Med* 1996; **335**: 1933–40.

Chapter 4

Prognosis in advanced heart failure

Richard Lehman

In Chapter 1, we noted the often erratic disease trajectory of heart failure and the frequency of sudden death – factors that would seem to make prediction in individual patients very difficult. The rather scanty data we have about doctors' predictions in heart failure would seem to bear this out. In early heart failure, primary care doctors may tend to overestimate the risk of death – at least in Switzerland.[1] On the other hand, the SUPPORT study,[2] carried out in the mid-1990s in the USA, found that 50% of heart failure patients were given a prognosis of more than 6 months on the day before they died.

Here we will look at some of the numerous factors that have been identified as helping to predict prognosis. There are well over a hundred in the literature, but we shall concentrate on those that are robust and easy to apply in a clinical context. There is no easily accessible review of prognosis in heart failure from the perspective of palliative care, so this chapter tries to deal with the whole picture, as well as with the specific tests and scoring systems that are of most use in predicting death in individual patients with advanced disease. Those who lack time or patience can go straight to the later sections to find these.

Throughout most of this section we are trying to use data from studies done on large series of patients to refine our predictions about the individual patient in front of us. This may seem quite a daunting task, but in the end we can fall back on a simple rule: *As a clinician, ask yourself 'would I be surprised if this patient were to die within the next year?'. If the answer is no, it is time to take a palliative care approach.* The purpose of this chapter is to help you determine more accurately which these patients are likely to be.

The evidence base for prognosis

Our knowledge of what determines outcome in heart failure comes from a number of sources. First, there are studies based in the community,[3-6] following up a large number of patients identified as having heart failure. Such studies have the great advantage of looking at a typical population with heart failure. Because diagnostic criteria vary, and disease registers may not be wholly accurate, such studies may be difficult to compare accurately, but they are still the most useful guide to what happens in primary care.

Second, there are studies based wholly or partly on follow-up of patients after a hospital admission for heart failure. Although these studies do not give an accurate picture of overall prognosis for all classes of heart failure in the community, they are still very useful in our quest for indicators of adverse outlook in individual patients. The Hillingdon study[7] can be included among these, because although it did its best to encourage direct recruitment from primary care, it ended up with a cohort drawn largely from hospital admissions for heart failure.

Third, there are data from the large interventional studies, such as those which established the role of ACE inhibitors and beta-adrenergic blockers in the past two decades. Unfortunately, the largest and best-known studies are recruited from hospital populations that are not comparable to the patients we typically encounter in the community – they are predominantly male, younger than average and were usually selected for the absence of some kinds of co-morbidity. The CHARM study[8] of 7,599 patients (69% male, mean age 66) has been very thoroughly analysed and is perhaps the best source of a risk score derived from history and common clinical variables, including cardiac, but not biochemical, investigations.

Lastly, and least typically, are patients undergoing selection for cardiac transplantation. They are mostly younger people with cardiomyopathy or very severe ischaemic damage. They are the most intensively studied group, and there is an extensive literature on physiological indicators which predict their likelihood of death. However, only fragments of this knowledge can be usefully applied to the patients we typically see in everyday clinical practice.

General indicators of prognosis

Here we are looking at general, easily assessed clinical features which give us an idea of how our patient is likely to fare. Later we will look at more sophisticated tests and scores.

Age

In the Rotterdam whole-population study,[3] the average age of heart failure patients was 77, and over five years their risk of death was 41% – a much lower mortality than in most hospital-recruited studies, but well above the age-matched population without heart failure, which was 15%. Every 10 years of age doubles the likelihood of death within four years in patients with heart failure. The Olmsted County study,[4] carried out at the same time in the USA, found exactly the same age distribution but a worse five-year prognosis (overall case-fatality 67%).

Hospital admission

In the Ontario study of patients discharged after a first admission for heart failure, case-fatality rates were much higher than in general population-based studies, at 40.1% at 12 months (rather than five years) in those over 75. For patients under 50 years it was 13.5%. In the Hillingdon study,[7] where 82% of the study population had been admitted to hospital for a first episode of heart failure, the overall case-fatality rate was similar, at 38% after 12 months.

It seems that heart failure sufficiently severe to warrant hospital admission has a much worse outlook than heart failure which can be managed entirely in primary care.

Gender

Women with a diagnosis of heart failure generally live longer than men: in one study (CIBIS-II),[9] the difference in mortality was 36%, although this may not be true of heart failure due to ischaemic heart disease.[9]

Aetiology

The aetiology of heart failure is changing with time, as rheumatic valvular disease is becoming rare, ischaemic heart disease is decreasing and more people are surviving to an age where their hearts become stiff for reasons which may not be clear-cut, but are probably related to preceding hypertension in most cases (see Chapter 2). Moreover, most patients with heart failure are now receiving drug therapy which prolongs life, so data like those from Framingham between 1948 and 1988[5] are now of purely historical value. Even the more recent Framingham data (1989–99)[6] may be misleading in the context of rapidly changing patterns of cardiovascular morbidity and therapy.

In general, however, the studies show that currently, heart failure due to known ischaemic disease has the worst prognosis.

Co-morbidity

Most patients with heart failure have other problems of old age (see Chapter 1), and these can markedly affect prognosis. Some of these co-morbidities may be due, at least in part, to the heart failure itself – this is probably true of depression, anaemia and cognitive impairment. Co-morbidities can be grouped together in scoring systems such as the Charlson Index, with twice the mortality in the highest scoring group as those with a zero score.

Diabetes

In community studies of heart failure, diabetes (mostly type 2) is typically found in 10–20% of patients. The data on the prognostic influence of diabetes are conflicting. Most studies find that diabetes has an adverse prognostic effect, and this is certainly true of heart failure accompanied by systolic dysfunction. However, diabetes can also be associated with diastolic heart failure, which has a better prognosis. The wide disparity between the various studies of prognosis in heart failure accompanied by diabetes may be explained by differences in case definition, stage of disease and ethnic mix.

Osteoarthritis

With an average age in the late 70s, the majority of heart failure patients are likely to have some degree of osteoarthritis. This features as an adverse prognostic factor in a large study from Toronto,[11] perhaps because these patients are more likely to be prescribed non-steroidal anti-inflammatory drugs. These become more dangerous as heart failure worsens and renal function declines.

Depression

Depression is common in heart failure, and in its later stages may be directly linked to cytokine release, causing depletion of serotonin. It is a markedly adverse prognostic factor,[12] but one which can probably be ameliorated by serotonin reuptake inhibitors.

Anaemia

Anaemia is a common precipitant of clinical heart failure, and often responds initially to iron supplementation. However, as discussed in Chapter 2, when heart failure progresses and renal impairment increases, erythropoietin production declines, leading to anaemia, which worsens breathlessness, impairs tissue oxygenation and is refractory to treatment. Thus anaemia becomes an increasingly adverse prognostic feature as heart failure worsens.[13]

Cognitive impairment

Cognitive impairment markedly worsens outlook in heart failure,[14] even outscoring cancer in some series. This may reflect a number of factors: dementia itself is linked with high mortality, independently of heart disease; patients with dementia may receive less intensive treatment, and they are likely to be less compliant with complex drug regimes. In some cases, apparent cognitive impairment may be directly due to depression – the 'depressive pseudo-dementia' syndrome. In end-stage heart failure, cognitive impairment may be due to complex factors affecting brain oxygenation, including anaemia, reduced cerebral blood supply and disordered breathing.

Pulmonary disease

Pulmonary disease is very common in elderly patients with heart failure, many of whom have smoked for most of their lives. Respiratory infection is also a common cause of decompensation and hospital admission in heart failure. These factors, added to the fact that heart failure is fundamentally a syndrome of impaired tissue oxygenation, make it remarkable that respiratory disease is not a more strongly adverse prognostic feature.

Cancer

Inevitably many elderly patients will have cancer as well as heart failure. To group all cancers together as 'malignancy', as in some studies, is of interest only to those looking at the approximate disease burden in the population. Each patient with cancer and heart failure will have an individual prognostic picture, as well as individual and complex needs.

Atrial fibrillation

Atrial fibrillation (AF) is common in heart failure, and new-onset AF often leads to sudden decompensation of previously stable heart failure. If this happens, the prognosis immediately worsens.[15]

Functional indicators

Remarkably, the patients with heart failure who are likely to survive longest are those we might think at highest risk – those who are overweight, have high blood pressure, high cholesterol and who drink alcohol. This has been labelled 'reverse epidemiology'.[16] So it is worth going through some of the data on various indicators of function in these patients, because it is not necessarily simply a matter of common sense.

Renal impairment

'Renal disease' is often listed as a co-morbidity in heart failure, but it is perhaps more helpful to regard it as an intrinsic functional consequence of advanced heart failure.[17] The physiological response to heart failure is, to an important extent, a response to decreased renal perfusion, but as we have seen in Chapter 2, the response actually worsens the problem and leads to the so-called 'cardio-renal syndrome', a vicious spiral of combined heart and kidney failure.

There may, of course, be other factors that worsen renal function. These include obstructive nephropathy in elderly men with prostatism, diabetic nephropathy and renal artery disease. Many of the drugs given for heart failure can worsen renal function initially, and lead to a rise in creatinine and a fall in sodium (*see* below).

Blood pressure

Most people with heart failure have been 'hypertensive' at some stage in their lives. But a damaged heart cannot maintain high pressures; and furthermore all treatment for heart failure lowers blood pressure. So, too, does the release of natriuretic peptides from overstretched atria and ventricles. Thus, once heart failure has set in, a low blood pressure is a marker for worsening disease and is associated with a poor prognosis.

Weight

Weight loss of more than 7.5% of previous normal weight over six months or more is associated with a very poor prognosis in heart failure.[18] This is the syndrome of cardiac cachexia, very similar to the cachexia of advanced cancer, and in common with it is probably driven by cytokines.

However, even if we remove bias by excluding any distorting effect from cardiac cachexia, there is still a generally favourable association between weight and survival in heart failure. This extends well into the range usually labelled 'obese'.[19]

Exercise capacity

Exercise capacity in heart failure shows little relation to systolic ejection fraction, but is linked to prognosis. This extends all the way from maximal exercise on a treadmill to pedometer measurements obtained from people who can barely walk. Some measurements techniques are discussed below.

Diuretic resistance

As part of the 'cardio-renal syndrome', patients become less responsive to loop diuretics, or patchily responsive so that they alternate between hypovolaemia and fluid overload. One retrospective analysis of an interventional trial has attempted to quantify diuretic response in relation to prognosis.[20] In normal clinical practice the best way to evaluate response is by trial of treatment and daily weighing: patients who need constant adjustment of their diuretics certainly have a poorer outlook.

Abnormal breathing

Heart failure is a state of chemoreceptor overdrive, so that patterns of respiration are abnormally sensitive to fluctuations in oxygen and carbon dioxide, and as a result breathing is inappropriately effortful. There is some evidence that reducing this overdrive by opioids is not only symptomatically beneficial but may be functionally beneficial too.

Many patients with heart failure exhibit an apnoeic (Cheyne-Stokes) pattern of breathing at night, which is of little prognostic importance. Cheyne-Stokes breathing by day, however, predicts death within a few months.[21]

Physiological measurements

Most physiological testing in heart failure is done in specialist units, usually either for research or for refining prognosis in younger patients who are being considered for surgery, including transplantation or left ventricular assist devices (LVADs). The following are some of the prognostically useful measurement techniques.

Peak O_2 uptake

The heart is required to produce a supply of oxygenated blood to all body systems under all normal conditions, including normal exertion. One way to measure how well the heart is functioning is to measure how much oxygen a patient can use up when exercising to the limit of their capacity. This has until recently been considered the 'gold standard' for prognosis, especially when used sequentially.[22] However, it requires highly specialised laboratory equipment and is therefore only normally used in research and in the evaluation of younger patients for surgery or transplantation.

Peak exercise cardiac power output

This test comes close to the 'gold standard' for determining the degree of physiological heart failure, but it is not widely available. It consists of measurements of cardiac output using carbon dioxide rebreathing techniques: the cardiac output is then multiplied by the mean arterial blood pressure to give the cardiac power output.[23] It proved of strong prognostic significance, although the study cohort – like most from hospital outpatients – was atypically young and male.

Daily activity level

At the opposite extreme from these complex laboratory-based measurements of 'pure' physiological parameters, we can use a simple instrument to measure what patients actually do in their everyday lives. One method is to attach a pedometer to measure the weekly walking distance. This is a powerful prognostic tool.[24]

Heart rate variability

As heart failure progresses, there is increasing autonomic dysfunction. This leads to a diminution in the ability of the cardiovascular system to accommodate to changing demands, and can be measured in several ways, the simplest of which is to do a 24-hour ambulatory electrocardiogram (ECG) and perform an automated analysis for heart rate variability. Patients at high risk of death from progressive heart failure[25] show the least heart rate variability, and this is also true for sudden death.[26]

Electrocardiographic changes

Almost all patients with heart failure have ECG abnormalities, and many detailed features of the ECG have been looked at for their prognostic significance. However, Q waves and AF are probably the only simple and widely available ECG parameters that clinicians use to help prediction in daily practice.

Restrictive filling pattern (echocardiographic)

Over recent years, there has been increasing interest in impaired ventricular filling as a contributor to the heart failure syndrome. Various methods of measurement have been proposed, and some of these are now robust enough to become part of routine echocardiographic assessment in patients with heart failure.

A restrictive filling pattern on Doppler echo is more closely related to prognosis than a decreased systolic ejection fraction.[27]

Systolic ejection fraction

The measurement of the proportion of blood pumped out by the ventricle at each beat (left ventricular systolic ejection fraction, LVSF) was used as the entry criterion for nearly all interventional heart failure trials from 1980 onwards, and this has bedevilled the subject ever since. It means that our evidence base is largely for heart failure with reduced LVSF, even though the LVSF has less predictive value than most parameters discussed in this section. However, it is reasonably easy to measure by various means, the least accurate of which is echocardiography, and it has some overall prognostic value.[28]

Specific markers

BUN/creatinine/uric acid

We have already seen that as part of the heart failure syndrome renal perfusion declines and neurohormonal overdrive ensues. As a result, the ability of the kidney to excrete nitrogenous waste products becomes impaired, and the plasma level of all these products – urea, uric acid and creatinine – goes up. In advanced heart failure there is also extra production of nitrogenous breakdown products from muscle catabolism. Studies of individual nitrogenous products such as uric acid[29] or total blood urea nitrogen (BUN)[30] have shown that increasing blood levels are associated with worsening prognosis.

Cystatin C

Nitrogenous waste products are not a very accurate indicator of renal function, and there has been recent interest in markers that correlate more closely to glomerular filtration rate (GFR). A promising candidate, not yet available for routine clinical use, is cystatin C, which is a protein continuously produced at a steady rate and freely filtered by the glomerulus. Serum levels of cystatin C have been shown to reflect GFR much more accurately than serum or plasma levels of creatinine. In a recent study, levels of cystatin C in patients with heart failure predicted cardiac events even in those with normal creatinine levels.[31]

Sodium

As heart failure worsens, the level of sodium in the blood falls for two reasons. One is the ever-increasing release of natriuretic (i.e. sodium-expelling) hormones from the heart; and the other is the increasing need to use sodium-depleting diuretics to relieve symptoms in advanced heart failure. Thus a fall in plasma sodium is a very useful and universally available surrogate measure for worsening heart failure.[32]

Troponins

One of the most significant advances in cardiology over the past decade has been the rapid adoption of cardiac troponin measurement as a way of detecting myocardial damage in acute coronary syndromes. The troponins are only released if there is myocardial cell injury, and we saw in an earlier chapter that in advanced heart failure, myocytes are injured and die in two ways – necrosis, which is usually due to acute ischaemia, or apoptosis, which can be caused by a number of mechanisms. In fact, there is probably an overlap between these mechanisms, and both may result in troponin release. In other words, troponin levels reflect a process of actual myocyte damage and loss in advanced heart failure. They are therefore of important prognostic value,[33] and troponin measurements are now routinely available in all acute hospitals.

B-type natriuretic peptide (BNP)

B-type or 'brain' natriuretic peptide is a potent hormone released by the ventricular myocytes in response to stretch or inflammation. Since heart failure involves both stretch and inflammation, it is impossible to have uncompensated heart failure without an elevation of BNP. The word natriuretic simply means 'promoting salt and water excretion', and we have seen that falling sodium can be used as a measure of hormonal activation in advancing heart failure.

So why not measure BNP directly? There are several ways of doing this, and whichever assay is chosen, the prognostic power is impressive – in fact greater than complex scoring systems based on the physiological parameters detailed above.[34] If we combine BNP with troponins, we can get even more predictive information.[35,36]

Thus, where it is available, BNP is the most useful measure of progression in heart failure, and predicts both progressive heart failure[37] and sudden death.[38]

There is no doubt that a single measurement of BNP is the simplest way of arriving at a prognosis in heart failure. In the future, BNP may be used to guide treatment in heart failure, and we will have much more data on the predictive value of sequential BNP levels in relation to therapy.

Scoring systems for prognosis

We have seen that there are numerous factors that a clinician can use in assessing which patients with heart failure may be getting closer to death. Of the biochemical markers, BNP shows outstanding promise. However, given that BNP measurement is not widely available in routine clinical practice, how can we best combine the information we have readily to hand in predicting what is going to happen to an individual patient?

One way is by using a validated score. There are a variety of such scores in heart failure, ranging from the NYHA classification, which is just a simple grading by breathlessness, to the very complex multifactorial scores used in heart transplantation clinics, such as the heart failure survival score (HFSS) or German Tansplant Society (GTS) score.[39] We shall look at a few scores that are validated for use in a community setting.

Table 4.1 Heart failure risk scoring system from the EFFECT study*

	No. of points	
Variable	30-day score[+]	1-year score[‡]
Years	+Age (in years)	+Age (in years)
Respiratory rate, min	+Rate (in breaths/min)	+Rate (in breaths/min)
(minimal 20; maxumum 45)[§]		
Systolic blood pressure, mm Hg[¶]		
≥ 180	−60	−50
160–179	−55	−45
140–159	−50	−40
120–139	−45	−35
100–119	−40	−30
90–99	−35	−25
<90	−30	−20
Urea nitrogen	+Level (in mg/dl)	+Level (in mg/dl)
(maximum, 60 mg/dl)[§**]		
Sodium concentration <136 mEq/l	+10	+10
Cerebrovascular disease	+10	+10
Dementia	+20	+15
Chronic obstructive pulmonary disease	+10	+10
Hepatic cirrhosis	+25	+35
Cancer	+15	+15
Haemoglobin <10.0 g/dl (<100 g/l)	NA	+10

NA, not applicable to 30-day model.
*An electronic version of the risk scoring system is available at:
www.ccort.ca/CHFriskmodel.asp
[+]Calculated as age + respiratory rate + systolic blood pressure + urea nitrogen + sodium points + cerebrovascular disease points + dementia points + chronic obstructive pulmonary disease points + hepatic cirrhosis points + cancer points.
[‡]Calculated as age + respiratory rate + systolic blood pressure + urea nitrogen + sodium points + cerebrovascular disease points + dementia points + chronic obstructive pulmonary disease points + hepatic cirrhosis points + cancer points + haemoglobin points.
[§]Values higher than maximum or lower than minimum are assigned the listed maximum or minimum values.
[¶]Increases were protective in both mortality models. Points are subtracted for higher blood pressure measurements.
[**]Maximum value is equivalent to 21 mmol/l. Score calculated using value in mg/dl.

Minnesota Living with Heart Failure questionnaire

As its name implies, this questionnaire was designed as a measurement tool for quality of life in heart failure, and has proved valuable in many studies for over a decade.[40] It has proved of prognostic value alongside BNP[41] and in addition to the Utrecht and EPICAL scores, of which details are given below.

EFFECT

The EFFECT (Enhanced Feedback for Effective Cardiac Treatment) study[11] was carried out in exemplary fashion by investigators based in Toronto who studied

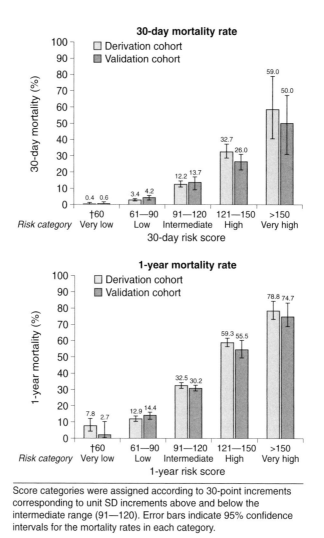

Figure 4.1 captions and data:

30-day mortality rate
- □ Derivation cohort
- ■ Validation cohort

Values: 0.4, 0.6 (†60 Very low); 3.4, 4.2 (61–90 Low); 12.2, 13.7 (91–120 Intermediate); 32.7, 26.0 (121–150 High); 59.0, 50.0 (>150 Very high)

Risk category / 30-day risk score

1-year mortality rate
- □ Derivation cohort
- ■ Validation cohort

Values: 7.8, 2.7 (†60 Very low); 12.9, 14.4 (61–90 Low); 32.5, 30.2 (91–120 Intermediate); 59.3, 55.5 (121–150 High); 78.8, 74.7 (>150 Very high)

Risk category / 1-year risk score

Score categories were assigned according to 30-point increments corresponding to unit SD increments above and below the intermediate range (91–120). Error bars indicate 95% confidence intervals for the mortality rates in each category.

Figure 4.1 Mortality rates stratified by 30-day and 1-year risk scores. From the EFFECT study, Lee *et al.* (2003).[11]

two cohorts of patients following a hospital admission for heart failure in order to generate and validate a prognostic scoring system based on Table 4.1. The predictive usefulness of the EFFECT scoring system is demonstrated in Figure 4.1.

Utrecht

A single cohort of patients from seven general hospitals in the Netherlands was studied in a similar way by investigators based in Utrecht.[42] A somewhat different set of parameters emerged, including absence of treatment with beta-blockers (Tables 4.2 and 4.3).

Table 4.2 Utrecht: regression coefficient and score of each predictor included in clinical model + drug treatment at baseline. With permission of BMJ Publishing Group from Bouvy et al.[42]

Predictor	Regression coefficient	Score*
Age (per year)	0.006	0.06
Male sex	0.42	+4
History of diabetes	0.86	+9
History of renal insufficiency	1.65	+17
Ankle oedema	1.03	+10
Weight (per kg)	−0.04	−0.4
Lower systolic or diastolic blood pressure†	0.74	+7
Absence of use of beta-blockers	1.30	+13

*The score per predictor is obtained by multiplying the regression coefficient by 10, and then rounded to nearest integer.
†Diastolic blood pressure <70 mm Hg or systolic blood pressure <110 mm Hg.

Table 4.3 Utrecht: distribution of patients according to the risk score derived from model 2. With permission of BMJ Publishing Group from Bouvy et al.[42]

Risk score	Total*	Incidence of mortality (%)†	Death‡	Survival‡
< −15	25	12.0	3	22
≥ −15 and < −5	29	10.3	3	26
≥ −5 and < −1	24	8.3	2	22
≥1 and <7	26	46.2	12	14
≥7 and <11	25	52	13	12
≥11	23	78.3	18	5
Total	152		51	101

Values represent absolute numbers of patients, except for incidence of mortality (%).
*Total number of patients per score category.
†Observed incidence of mortality per score category.
‡Number of patients who died and survived per score category.

EPICAL

The EPICAL study (Epidémiologie de l'Insuffisance Cardiaque Avancée en Lorraine)[32,43] identified patients with NYHA class III/IV who had been admitted to hospital. The prognostic scoring system which it generated is relatively simple and is summarised in Figure 4.2. This applies primarily to patients with known ischaemia: the papers also give a slightly different set of criteria that can be applied to those with non-ischaemic cardiomypathy.

CHART

CHART is a Japanese prospective observational study of chronic heart failure,

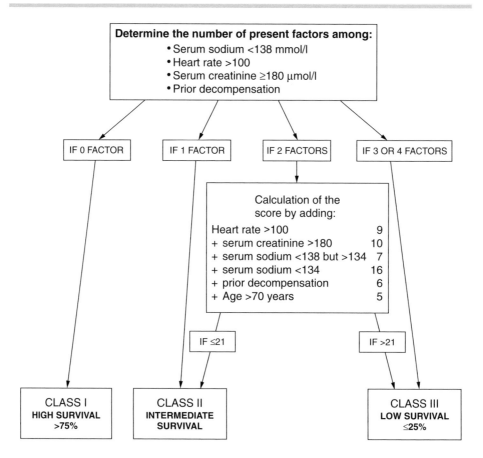

Figure 4.2 EPICAL: a clinical scoring system for heart failure due to ischaemic heart disease. With permission of Elsevier from Alla *et al.* (2000).[32]

which has so far reported only on sudden death as an outcome.[44] The following parameters were found to carry an approximately two-fold risk of sudden death:

- non-sustained ventricular tachycardia
- ejection fraction <30%
- left ventricular end-diastolic diameter >60 mm
- BNP >200 pg/ml
- diabetes.

Those with three or more of the above had a hazard ratio for sudden death of 9, equating to a three-year risk of about 30%.

It has to be recognised that although scores of many kinds have been developed for most chronic diseases, most are rarely used by clinicians in everyday practice. However, a basic computer-generated prognostic score for heart failure would be very easy to use in most settings, especially heart failure clinics. Research needs to be done to validate such a score for patients in the last year of life in a community setting. Unlike most existing scores, it would necessarily incorporate BNP.

Summary

Heart failure is changing from being an unpredictable condition to one for which there is now a range of easily used prognostic tools. There is a need for further work in the community to validate scores incorporating BNP. However, the basic question we need to ask ourselves remains: *Would I be surprised if this patient were to die within the next year, and should I adopt a palliative care approach?*

This is a question we need to ask about every patient who has had a hospital admission for heart failure. In fact, we need to go further when we see the discharge summary of a patient who has been admitted with decompensated heart failure, and ask ourselves: *Is there any reason why I should* not *start thinking about supportive care for this patient?*

The risk is that, given the difficulties with prognosis in heart failure, clinicians become paralysed in their ability to do anything other than proceed relentlessly with treatments directed at the heart failure alone, rather than seeing the effects on many areas of the patient's life that require help. A problem-oriented approach enables a patient to have access to appropriate services when needed, rather than withholding this because 'we're not at that stage yet'. Better prognostic indicators will help in this process, but the fundamental focus should always be on the needs of the individual patient.

References

1   Muntwyler J, Abetel G, Gruner C, Follath F. One-year mortality among unselected out-patients with heart failure. *Eur Heart J* 2002; **23**: 1861–6.

2   Levenson JW, McCarthy EP, Lynn J, Davis RB, Phillips RS. The last six months of life for patients with congestive heart failure. *J Am Geriatr Soc* 2000; **48**(Suppl 5): S101–9.

3   Mosterd A, Cost B, Hoes AW, de Bruijne MC, Deckers JW, Hofman A, Grobbee DE. The prognosis of heart failure in the general population. *Eur Heart J* 2001; **22**: 1318–27.

4   Senni M, Tribouilloy CM, Rodeheffer RJ, Jacobsen SJ, Evans JM, Bailey KR, Redfield MM. Congestive heart failure in the community: trends in incidence and survival in a 10-year period. *Arch Intern Med* 1999; **159**: 29–34.

5   Kalon KL, Anderson KM, Kannel WB, Grossman W, Levy D. Survival after the onset of congestive heart failure in Framingham Heart Study subjects. *Circulation* 1993; **88**: 107–15.

6   Levy D, Kenchaiah S, Larson MG, Benjamin E *et al.* Long-term trends in the incidence of and survival with heart failure. *New Eng J Med* 2002; **347**: 1397–402.

7   Cowie MR, Wood DA, Coats AJS, Thompson SG, Suresh V, Poole-Wilson PA, Sutton GC. Survival of patients with a new diagnosis of heart failure: a population based study. *Heart* 2000; **83**: 505–10.

8   Pocock SJ, Wang D, Pfeffer MA *et al.* Predictors of mortality and morbidity in patients with chronic heart failure. *Eur Heart J* 2006; **27**: 65–75.

9   Simon T, Mary-Krause M, Funck-Brentano C, Jaillon P. Sex differences in the prognosis of congestive cardiac failure: results from the Cardiac Insufficiency Bisoprolol Study (CIBIS II). *Circulation* 2001; **103**: 375–80.

10 Ghali JK, Krause-Steinrauf HJ, Adams KF *et al.* Gender differences in advanced heart failure: insights from the BEST study. *J Am Coll Cardiol* 2003; **42**: 2128–34.

11 Lee DS, Austin PC, Rouleau JL, Liu PP *et al.* Predicting mortality among patients

hospitalized for heart failure: derivation and validation of a clinical model. *JAMA* 2003; **290**: 2581–7.

12 Rumsfeld JS, Havranek E, Masoudi FA, Peterson ED, Jones P, Too JF, Krumholz HM, Spertus JA. Depressive symptoms are the strongest predictors of short-term declines in health status in patients with heart failure. *J Am Coll Cardiol* 2003; **42**: 1811–17.

13 Mozaffarian D, Nye R, Levy WC. Anemia predicts mortality in severe heart failure. The prospective randomized amlodipine survival evaluation (PRAISE). *J Am Coll Cardiol* 2003; **41**: 1933–9.

14 Zucalla G, Pedone C, Cesari M, Pahor M, Marzetti E *et al.* The effect of cognitive impairment on mortality among hospitalized patients with heart failure. *Am J Med* 2003; **115**: 97–103.

15 Wang TJ, Larson MG, Levy D, Vasan RS, Leip EP *et al.* Temporal relations of atrial fibrillation and congestive heart failure and their joint influence on mortality: the Framingham Heart Study. *Circulation* 2003; **107**: 2920–5.

16 Kalantar-Zadeh K, Block G, Horwich T, Fonarow GC. Reverse epidemiology of conventional cardiovascular risk factors in patients with chronic heart failure. *J Am Coll Cardiol* 2004; **43**: 1439–44.

17 Gottlieb SS, Abraham W, Butler J, Forman DE, Loh E *et al.* The prognostic importance of different definitions of worsening renal function in congestive heart failure. *J Card Fail* 2002; **8**:136–41.

18 Anker SD, Ponikowski P, Varney S, Chua TP, Clark AL *et al.* Wasting as an independent risk factor for mortality in chronic heart failure. *Lancet* 1997; **349**: 1050–3.

19 Lavie CJ, Osman AF, Milani RV, Mehra MR. Body composition and prognosis in chronic systolic heart failure: the obesity paradox. *Am J Cardiol* 2003; **91**: 891–4.

20 Neuberg GW, Miller AB, O'Connor CM, Belkin RN, Carson PE *et al.* Diuretic resistance predicts mortality in patients with advanced heart failure. *Am Heart J* 2002; **144**: 31–8.

21 Andreas S, Hagenah G, Moller C, Werner GS, Kreuzer H. Cheyne-Stokes respiration and prognosis in congestive heart failure. *Am J Cardiol* 1996; **78**: 1260–4.

22 Lavie CJ, Milani RV, Mehra MR. Peak exercise oxygen pulse and prognosis in chronic heart failure. *Am J Cardiol* 2004; **93**: 588–93.

23 Williams SG, Cooke GA, Wright DJ, Parsons WJ, Riley RL, Marshall P, Tan L-B. Peak exercise cardiac power output: a direct indicator of cardiac function strongly predictive of prognosis in chronic heart failure. *Eur Heart J* 2001; **22**: 1496–503.

24 Walsh JT, Charlesworth A, Andrews R, Hawkins M, Cowley AJ. Relation of daily activity levels in patients with chronic heart failure to long-term prognosis. *Am J Cardiol* 1997; **79**: 1364–9.

25 Nolan J, Batin PD, Andrews R, Lindsay SJ *et al.* Prospective study of heart rate variability and mortality in chronic heart failure (UK-Heart). *Circulation* 1998; **98**: 1510–16.

26 La Rovere MT, Pinna GD, Maestri R, Mortara A *et al.* Short-term heart rate variability strongly predicts sudden cardiac death in chronic heart failure patients. *Circulation* 2003; **107**: 565–70.

27 Tabet J-Y, Logeart D, Geyer C, Guiti C, Ennezat PV, Dahan M, Cohen-Solal A. Comparison of the prognostic value of left ventricular filling and peak oxygen uptake in patients with systolic heart failure. *Eur Heart J* 2000; **21**: 1864–71.

28 Florea VG, Hencin MY, Cioira M, Anker SD, Doehner W *et al.* Echocardiographic determinants of mortality in patients >67 years of age with chronic heart failure. *Am J Cardiol* 2000; **86**: 158–61.

29 Kerzner R, Gage BF, Freedland KE, Rich MW. Predictors of mortality in younger and older patients with heart failure and preserved or reduced left ventricular ejection fraction. *Am Heart J* 2003; **146**: 286–90.

30 Anker SD, Doehner W, Rauchhaus M, Sharma R *et al.* Uric acid and survival in chronic

heart failure: validation and application in metabolic, functional, and haemodynamic staging. *Circulation* 2003; **107**: 1991–7.

31 Arimoto T, Takeishi Y, Niizeki T, Takabatake N *et al.* Cystatin C, a novel measure of renal function, is an independent predictor of cardiac events in patients with heart failure. *J Card Fail* 2005; **11**: 595–601.

32 Alla F, Briançon S, Jullière Y, Mertes P-M, Villemot J-P, Zannad F. Differential clinical prognostic classifications in dilated and ischemic advanced heart failure: the EPICAL study. *Am Heart J* 2000; **139**: 895–904.

33 Horwich TB, Patel J, MacLellan WR, Fonarow GC. Cardiac troponin I is associated with impaired hemodynamics in progressive left ventricular dysfunction, and increased mortality rates in advanced heart failure. *Circulation* 2003; **108**: 833–8.

34 Koglin J, Pehlivanli S, Schwaiblmair M, Vogeser M, Cremer P, von Scheidt W. Role of brain natriuretic peptide in risk stratification of patients with congestive heart failure. *J Am Coll Cardiol* 2001; **38**: 1934–41.

35 Ralli S, Horwich TB, Fonarow GC. Relationship between anemia, cardiac troponin 1, and B-type natriuretic peptide levels and mortality in patients with advanced heart failure. *Am Heart J* 2005; **150**: 1220–7.

36 Fonarow GC, Horwich TB. Combining natriuretic peptides and necrosis markers in determining prognosis in heart failure. *Rev Cardiovasc Med* 2003; **4**(Suppl 4): S20–8.

37 Gardner RS, Ozalp F, Murday AJ, Robb SD, McDonagh TA. N-terminal pro-brain natriuretic peptide. A new gold standard in predicting mortality in patients with advanced heart failure. *Eur Heart J* 2003; **24**: 1735–43.

38 Berger R, Strecker K, Huelsmann M, Moser P, Frey B, Bojic A, Stanek B, Pacher R. B-type natriuretic peptide predicts sudden death in patients with chronic heart failure. *Circulation* 2002; **105**: 2392–7.

39 Smits JM, Deng MC, Hummel M, De Meester J *et al.* A total prognostic model for predicting waiting-list mortality for a total national cohort of adult heart-transplant candidates. *Transplantation* 2003; **76**: 1185–9.

40 Guyatt M. Measurement of health-related quality of life in heart failure. *J Am Coll Cardiol* 1993; **22**(4 Suppl A); 185A–191A.

41 Hulsmann M, Berger R, Sturm B, Bojic A, Woloszczuk W, Bergler K-J, Pacher R. Prediction of outcome by neurohormonal activation, the six-minute walk test and the Minnesota Living with Heart Failure Questionnaire in an outpatient cohort with congestive heart failure. *Eur Heart J* 2002; **23**: 886–91.

42 Bouvy ML, Heerdink ER, Leufkens HG, Hoes AW. Predicting mortality in patients with heart failure: a pragmatic approach. *Heart* 2003; **89**: 605–9.

43 Alla F, Briançon S, Guillemin F, Juillière Y, Mertes PM, Villemot JP, Zannad F; EPICAL Investigators. Self-rating of quality of life provides additional prognostic information in heart failure: insights into the EPICAL study. *Eur J Heart Fail* 2002; **4**: 337–43.

44 Watanabe J, Shinozaki T, Shiba N, Fukahori K *et al.* Accumulation of risk markers predicts the incidence of sudden death in patients with chronic heart failure. *Eur J Heart Fail* 2006; **8**: 237–42.

Chapter 5

Symptom relief for advanced heart failure

Miriam Johnson and Louise Gibbs

Achieving symptom relief in advanced heart failure is a challenging task. There is a negligible basis of specific research on which to base treatment. Even the clinical experience that has been anecdotally reported is sparse. There is, however, a wealth of evidence about symptom relief in other illnesses, most notably cancer, that gives a basic framework from which to start.[1]

The first principle is comprehensive symptom assessment, which is part of a global assessment of physical, psychological, social and spiritual need. This assessment should include a thorough history, plus appropriate examination and investigations. The core of the management plan should be explanation and discussion. General and specific treatments should be planned proactively and reviewed regularly. Reversible or underlying causes of symptoms should be treated wherever possible. Issues such as polypharmacy and compliance are important, and the use of self-medication charts and pre-filled weekly drug systems such as dosette boxes may help. For the purposes of this book, the focus is on the physical aspects in this chapter, and the psychosocial and spiritual aspects in the next. In practice, of course, there is no such artificial division.

Symptoms

The main symptoms discussed in the clinic or surgery will be the classic triad of breathlessness, fatigue and peripheral swelling, which may involve ascites as well as lower-limb oedema. Indeed, the severity of breathlessness forms the basis of the NYHA classification. However, further enquiry often reveals a multitude of physical concerns from the patient, including constipation, dry mouth, anorexia, weight loss, nausea, insomnia and a variety of pains. Confusion and memory loss may be subtle and easily missed. Symptoms may be in part due to psychological problems such as anxiety and low mood, which are discussed elsewhere in the book but must be considered as part of a symptom assessment. Symptoms currently remain unrecognised and unalleviated in the months or even years prior to death in a quarter to a third of patients.[2] The challenge is to consider them as a central part of the clinical syndrome of heart failure and actively manage them accordingly.

Patient preference regarding outcome of treatment has been a neglected area.[3] A full understanding of individual preferences for symptom improvement versus survival will have important management implications for each patient.[3,4]

Discussing these issues with patients requires good communication skills and many clinicians find this difficult. Hence many patients still do not have their diagnosis, prognosis or treatment preferences discussed openly, which can make optimum symptom control hard to achieve. Most heart failure patients are treated by a number of doctors as they approach the end of life, especially if they have repeated hospital admissions. There is a potential for conflict between the aims of maximising life-prolonging treatment and respecting the patient's possible wish to prioritise symptom control. Different professionals may also have differing views on issues such as physical activity, diet and fluid intake. There is great potential for confusion about changes of drug treatment and for hazardous polypharmacy.

Even in patients receiving optimal management, the symptom burden can be considerable. Anderson *et al*. assessed 66 patients attending a heart failure clinic and compared their concerns with 213 palliative care patients.[5] A high number of symptoms were reported in both groups, but those with heart failure had less support from district nurses, hospice, social work or physiotherapy. Heart failure patients said dyspnoea (55%), angina (32%) and tiredness (27%) were the *most* troublesome symptoms, and tiredness was reported by 82%. Documented action was greater for physical than for other problems, but overall was less for heart failure patients than for those from the palliative care clinic. Studies by Murray *et al*. comparing patients with lung cancer and those with heart failure, and a study looking at needs of heart failure patients admitted in west London confirm the same picture.[6,7] The unpalatable conclusion is that heart failure patients have needs that are not being met, and they are disadvantaged compared with those designated with 'palliative care' needs.

Optimisation of medical management

It is very important that a patient is taking optimum tolerated medical treatment (*see* Chapter 3), as it is clear that good symptom control is based on this. Therefore a shared care approach between cardiology and palliative and primary care is adopted, and access to cardiology advice is maintained throughout the illness. The balance and emphasis may alter as the patient's disease progresses, but this underlying message remains the same. Even in the dying phase (*see* Chapter 8) patients are likely to need a loop diuretic and perhaps nitrates (furosemide given subcutaneously and nitrates transdermally when the intravenous route becomes difficult or inappropriate) to control breathlessness and angina in addition to the 'standard' opioid, benzodiazepine, anti-emetic and anti-secretory medication.

There is clear evidence that many patients with heart failure are suboptimally managed in terms of the evidence-based therapies such as ACE inhibitors, beta-blockers and spironolactone.[8,9] The situation is exacerbated by the common problems of each admission being under the care of a different physician, with seemingly no one grasping an overview of the clinical progression, and of poor monitoring that fails to sustain improvements made. Fluid status (sometimes helped by defining the 'dry weight' of a person) and renal function require monitoring, and diuretics often require frequent adjustment. It is hoped that the growth of interested individual clinicians (in both primary and secondary care) and a spectrum of specialist services will improve this situation. Any individual's management plan needs to include not only cognition, compliance and poly-pharmacy issues, but also the challenges presented by co-morbidities. More than half of patients will have one or a combination of co-morbidities such as peripheral vascular disease, chronic obstructive pulmonary disease (COPD), diabetes, arthritis, renal failure and depression. Clearly, professionals not only need to be aware of each other, but also need to work together. The general practitioner can find themself bombarded with conflicting advice from specialist physicians as well as specialist nurses, and some of this advice may already have been conveyed to the patient, creating fertile ground for misunderstanding and loss of confidence.

For these reasons some specialist palliative care workers feel unsure about getting involved, concerned that they will not have the skills to manage these medications. However, there have been joint approaches across the UK in the form of shared-care models, with patients (and carers) benefiting from both teams (*see* Chapter 10). In some cases, all heart failure monitoring and disease management is done by generalists and cardiac specialists, with specialist palliative care advising as an 'add-on' service. In others, specialist palliative care has, through joint working and education, taken over some of these roles, learning the necessary skills and buying the necessary weighing scales.

Therapeutic options for improved symptom control

Table 5.1 gives a brief list of practical tips for symptom control in heart failure.

Breathlessness

Breathlessness is one of the most serious concerns, from the terrifying experience of paroxysmal nocturnal dyspnoea to the debilitating breathlessness on exertion. It is closely allied to muscle weakness and fatigue, and even patients who are at dry weight may experience limiting breathlessness.

Assessment

Potentially reversible factors should be looked for and treated. For example, persistent pleural effusion despite diuretics may need drainage, and chest infections should be treated with antibiotics. A chest X-ray may be useful. Most patients with heart failure have a history of smoking and may well have coexistent obstructive airways disease or may even develop bronchogenic carcinoma. It is important to look for and manage associated anxiety, as panic may be a significant exacerbating factor. Ascites and an engorged liver can restrict diaphragmatic movement and inspiration.

General measures

Evidence from work done in lung cancer patients suggests that a range of non-pharmacological interventions can ameliorate intractable breathlessness.[10] Although there is no published evidence to date in heart failure patients, some such pulmonary rehabilitation services, both in hospitals and hospices, are including heart failure patients in their programmes. A broad approach will include

Table 5.1 Tips for symptom control in heart failure

Symptom	Simple symptom control options
Breathlessness	Optimally treat heart failure and co-morbid diseases, including anxiety 'Pulmonary rehabilitation' Opioids: • oral morphine 2.5–5 mg four hourly and titrate • manage common opioid side effects • seek advice if renal function poor or opioid toxicity
Fatigue	Search for reversible factors Consider treatment of anaemia Appropriate exercise Avoid steroids and progestagens
Pain	Avoid NSAIDs and tricyclic antidepressants Use the WHO analgesic ladder: follow step 1, then 2, then 3 (all drugs oral) • Step 1: paracetamol 1 g qds, caplets or tablets • Step 2: paracetamol 500 mg + codeine 30 mg, 2 tablets qds or tramadol 50–100 mg qds +/− regular paracetamol • Step 3: morphine 5–10 mg four hourly and prn; titrate every 48 hours if pain not controlled • manage common opioid side effects • seek advice if renal function poor, opioid toxicity or good pain control not achieved
Nausea and vomiting	Search for reversible factors Oral metoclopramide 10–20 mg tds or haloperidol 1.5–3 mg od; avoid cyclizine
Constipation	Laxative: • softener/surfactant: lactulose, polyethylene glycol or sodium docusate +/− • stimulant: senna
Dry mouth	Avoid acids Mucin-based saliva substitutes, sugar-free chewing gum
Skin problems	Aqueous cream as soap substitute and moisturiser 2% menthol in aqueous cream for itch
Depression	Have a low index of suspicion for depression Consider non-drug approaches Avoid tricyclic antidepressants and drugs with many potential drug interactions (e.g. fluoxetine) Sertraline 50 mg od, citalopram 10–20 mg od, mirtazapine 15–30 mg od

understanding the meaning of breathlessness for the individual, breathing exercises to train for more effective respiration for those with dysfunctional breathing patterns, assisting adaptation to better ways of coping with associated fear and panic through relaxation techniques, pacing of activities and even simple use of a fan.

Restrictive undergarments are still discovered on occasion, particularly in the elderly; persuading the patient to discard these may help.

The potential benefit from a thorough social and practical needs review, with referral on to therapy, welfare and social services as appropriate, cannot be overstated and is discussed more fully in Chapter 6.

Specific measures

Opioids

Morphine has been used empirically for many years to relieve symptoms in acute left ventricular failure or myocardial ischaemia, or when it is perceived that there is 'nothing else we can do' and the patient will die imminently. There is reluctance to use it chronically for symptom relief in patients who are not actively dying, but nevertheless are very restricted by breathlessness, for fear of respiratory depression and lack of published evidence.[11,12] Regular opioids are a potentially useful palliative therapy, postulated to act through reduction in chemoreceptor hypersensitivity and subsequent improvement in the abnormal ventilatory patterns found in heart failure.[13,14] Haemodynamic effects are not thought to be important.[15]

In heart failure, the published literature comprises one report of two cases of nebulised morphine, two single-dose studies and more recently a pilot study investigating the use of regular chronic dosing with oral morphine for the relief of breathlessness.[15–18] One single-dose study looked at the effect of dihydrocodeine on exercise tolerance and chemosensitivity, and the other study looked at the effect on exercise tolerance of a small dose of diamorphine prior to the exercise. The results of both studies demonstrated an improvement in abnormal ventilatory patterns. The pilot study was a double-blinded, randomised placebo controlled cross-over study of 10 patients with NYHA class III/IV heart failure.[16] On morphine, median breathlessness score (Visual Analogue Score 0–100 mm) fell by 23 mm ($p = 0.022$) by day 2. The improvement in breathlessness score was maintained throughout the active arm of the study. Side effects of sedation, constipation and nausea were minimal. Sedation scores increased until day 3, but started to improve again on day 4. Four patients reported constipation on morphine compared with only one on placebo, but there were no differences between the two arms in nausea. Importantly, no differences between the two arms were seen in blood pressure, pulse or respiratory rate, indicating that, in closely monitored appropriate patients, the high level of safety concerns may be unfounded. In the active arm, a dose of 5 mg oral morphine four times a day was used. This dose was reduced in renal dysfunction. Patients with a serum creatinine of 300 µmol/l or more were excluded. Six patients identified morphine rather than placebo as having helped their breathlessness and, one year after study completion, four continued to take morphine regularly with continued benefit.

Thus chronically administered oral morphine gave clinically significant improvement in breathlessness and tolerability was good. Further studies are needed, answering questions such as appropriate patient selection and choice and dosing regime of opioid (particularly in COPD or renal impairment).

Oxygen

Oxygen therapy is considered part of the first-line management of acute left heart failure in addition to diuretics and opioids. However, for heart failure patients, recommendations do not routinely include oxygen therapy. Arterial desaturation and hypoxia on exercise are not common in patients with compensated heart failure. Studies investigating the effect of increased inspired oxygen concentrations on exercise duration and subjective dyspnoea have produced conflicting, but mainly negative, results.[18–20] There have been no studies looking specifically at the benefits of oxygen on the sensation of breathlessness in severe heart failure.

Lung disease is common in many patients with heart failure and these patients may gain some symptomatic benefit with oxygen therapy because of that. Thus decisions need to be made on an individual patient basis taking into account all factors.[21] The practicalities of providing ambulatory oxygen should be remembered in considering cost-benefit balance in addition to the psychological dependence that can occur for such patients. Some patients become psychologically dependent on oxygen therapy even when it is of doubtful benefit, creating panic if there is a problem with supply.

Benzodiazepines

The use of benzodiazepines (as required and regularly) in the symptomatic palliation of breathlessness is widespread in cancer palliative care practice. There is little hard evidence for this practice. Fears of dangerous respiratory depression may not be borne out in clinical practice, but there are potentially serious problems of memory loss, falls, tolerance and addiction with chronic use, particularly in the frail elderly. Patients with significant anxiety, depression or panic attacks (when breathlessness spirals out of control) should first be treated with the specific breathing control and relaxation techniques of pulmonary rehabilitation or cognitive approaches such as cognitive behavioural therapy, and if drug treatment is needed, anxiolytic antidepressants such as mirtazapine and selective serotonin re-uptake inhibitors such as citalopram, which are known to be safe in heart failure, can be used. In appropriate cases, judicious use of an intermediate-acting benzodiazepine such as lorazepam or lormetazepam to gain control of panic, in addition to the above, may be useful. Lorazepam tablets can in fact be quickly absorbed sublingually.

Fatigue

Fatigue is the other major complaint of patients with chronic heart failure, and can be difficult to improve. Again, the principle of a full assessment, looking for reversible factors is important. Table 5.2 lists the common ones. Timing and amount of diuretics can impinge on quality of sleep, and indeed sleep disorder due to other reasons can all impact on daytime wakefulness. Sleep apnoea and nocturnal hypoventilation are important to diagnose, as some patients gain benefit from non-invasive ventilation at night. Complaints of morning headache and daytime somnolence from the patient should prompt questioning of the sleep partner (if there is one).

Anaemia of chronic disease (normochromic, normocytic) is often seen in advanced heart failure, and indicates the severity of disease. Silverberg *et al.* treated 40 octogenarians with resistant severe heart failure and anaemia (Hb <12 g/dl) with subcutaneous erythropoietin and intravenous iron.[22] Patients had a marked improvement in cardiac function, breathlessness and fatigue. Hospital admissions were reduced and renal function stabilised. The authors suggested that anaemia was not only a marker for disease severity, but itself aggravated the

Table 5.2 Fatigue in heart failure: common potentially reversible factors

Diuretics	Over-diuresis
	Hypokalaemia
Beta-blockers	Tiredness
Sleep disorders	Orthopnoea, paroxysmal dyspnoea, sleep apnoea and nocturnal hypoventilation
Depression	
Anaemia	
Exercise deconditioning	

progression of heart failure. However, for many patients this approach may be considered invasive, and more research is required to evaluate the cost-effectiveness of this expensive treatment.

It has become increasingly accepted that muscle bulk and function play a very important role in the symptoms of heart failure and that exercise is beneficial. Exercise programmes appear to be safe in stable chronic heart failure.[23] Exercise training and the physiotherapy and rehabilitation programmes appear to be a very important part of optimal management. Survival may be improved[23] and symptoms such as fatigue and breathlessness improved by even low-level exercise programmes.[24,25] Patients may need reassurance and encouragement as they may be very nervous of physical exercise and worry that it may cause further cardiac events.

Prioritisation and pacing of activities can be very helpful; many patients need assistance to adjust to their limitations, so that they become less frustrating. Without such help, heart failure patients can become stuck in a cycle of physical inactivity and progressive limitation, which can contribute to depression and social isolation.

Pain

Pain is an often under-recognised symptom in heart failure. Multiple studies have shown it to be prevalent, severe and prolonged. Pain can be cardiac (angina pectoris) and non-cardiac (musculoskeletal pain, dyspepsia, gout, peripheral vascular disease, from oedematous legs or tense ascites). Assessment and management of pain needs to follow the basic principles laid out at the beginning of this chapter.

Non-cardiac pain

The management of chronic pain, both in malignant and non-malignant disease, requires regular administration of analgesics, up-titrated to achieve effective pain control. A combination of drugs with different actions is often required. The World Health Organization (WHO) three-step analgesic ladder provides an excellent framework with which to start (Table 5.3).[26] Step 1 is paracetamol, which should be given regularly at a dose of 1 g four times a day. Step 2 is to add or substitute a weak opioid, such as codeine, dihydrocodeine or tramadol. Fixed combination tablets of weak opioid and paracetamol can be useful aids to acceptability and compliance, but those with a subtherapeutic dose of opioid should be avoided, i.e. use paracetamol 500 mg + codeine 30 mg, two tablets four times a day. If this

Table 5.3 WHO analgesic ladder

Step 1 Mild pain	Non-opioid +/− adjuvant	E.g. paracetamol 1 g qds
Step 2 Moderate pain	Mild opioid + non-opioid +/− adjuvant	E.g. co-codamol 30/500 mg two qds
Step 3 Severe pain	Strong opioid +/− adjuvant	E.g. morphine given regularly, dose titrated to individual patient need

is ineffective, do not swap to another weak opioid, but move up to the next step. Step 3 is for strong opioids. Sometimes paracetamol will still have an additive effect on pain and can be continued. Weak opioids should be stopped when strong opioids are started. Oral morphine remains the strong opioid of choice, although as it is renally excreted, additional care must be taken in the presence of renal dysfunction. Morphine can be taken as an immediate-release tablet or liquid regularly four hourly or as a modified-release preparation. Both 12-hourly and 24-hourly preparations are available in the UK. Immediate-release morphine is often used initially to titrate to the dose required, and the patient is then transferred to a modified-release preparation. Once stable, immediate-release morphine must still be prescribed to be taken for any breakthrough pain, the dose being one sixth of the total 24-hour dose. Patients who have been on the maximum dose of a weak opioid such as codeine 60 mg four times a day will usually require at least oral morphine 10 mg four hourly on transfer to step 3. Use 5 mg four hourly if patient, carer or clinician is not confident in morphine's use, but be prepared to up-titrate quickly.

Common side effects of opioids (weak and strong) should be anticipated and treated. Most patients get constipated and need regular laxatives. Initial nausea occurs in about a third of patients, who should be prescribed an anti-emetic such as metoclopramide. Drowsiness should wear off after two to three days, but will often recur at each up-titration. Affected patients should be counselled not to drive when thus affected, but there are no specific driving restrictions in patients who are not drowsy on stable morphine. The use of alternative strong opioids is beyond the scope of this text. Their use will usually require advice from clinicians familiar with them, such as those from specialist palliative care.

Non-aspirin, non-steroidal anti-inflammatory drugs (NSAIDs) are contra-indicated in heart failure patients because of their fluid-retaining side effects. By expanding the intravascular volume, NSAIDs also blunt the response to diuretics. One study has shown a doubling of the risk of hospital admission for worsening heart failure in previously stable patients who were started on an NSAID. There were no differences between NSAIDs and no dose response was observed. The risk of admission was highest within the first few days of initiation, and usually happened within 30 days.[27] The risk of gastrointestinal bleeding is also greater in patients with significant co-morbidity such as heart failure. Many of these patients also have renal dysfunction, or are on a combination of loop diuretic and ACE inhibitor – adding an NSAID to this cocktail is potentially nephrotoxic, particularly in the elderly. It is therefore recommended that *all* NSAIDs be avoided in heart failure patients if at all possible. If there is no other option for pain control then careful monitoring of weight, renal function and symptoms is mandatory in anything other than a pre-terminal situation.

Restricting the use of NSAIDs can make management of arthritis difficult, but not impossible, as application of the WHO analgesic ladder is appropriate and applicable. Treatment of gout can be managed with colchicine, although almost all patients develop diarrhoea within 48 hours of the dose required. This can be disastrous in patients with poor mobility and may result in the humiliation of faecal incontinence.

Some pains do not respond fully to 'conventional' analgesics. Neuropathic pain is the classic example, but in practice this is also true of the pain of tender, sore legs in heart failure. Adjuvant analgesics are usually required. Tricyclic antidepressants have a better profile of effectiveness and side effects than anticonvulsants, but tricyclics are relatively contraindicated in heart failure because of their anticholinergic activity. Thus an anticonvulsant such as gabapentin is safest in heart failure. Again, its use will usually require advice from clinicians familiar with it such as those from specialist palliative care.

Cardiac pain

The pain from angina pectoris is usually controlled with anti-anginal medication, but there are patients for whom this remains a severe and limiting problem despite optimal treatment. Intravenous diamorphine is well accepted in the relief of acute ischaemic cardiac pain. However, although morphine is effective in chronic pain there is a reluctance to use it, partly again because of a paucity of literature confirming efficacy and safety. Recently, a small prospective study of 12 patients attending a regional refractory angina clinic demonstrated successful titration of sustained-release preparations of morphine or oxycodone (for those with unacceptable drowsiness or pruritus).[28] These patients had failed to respond to psychological therapies, transcutaneous nerve stimulation (TENS) and temporary sympathetic blockade. Patients were followed up for 12 weeks. Only two patients were unable to tolerate opioids because of sedation and nausea. Frequency of angina and total pain burden was reduced, with a corresponding increase in exercise capacity, general health and vitality. Significantly, an improvement was also seen in depression score and social functioning, highlighting the impact of chronic physical symptoms. Opioids were well tolerated and low risk in these patients in this setting. Again, all we have to date is a small study, and more research is urgently needed so that the use of an effective drug can become more acceptable to clinician and patient alike.

TENS is also used with some success in intractable angina, but its use has not become commonplace. Studies are difficult to conduct (hard to blind treatment) and the placebo effect is high. However, reports suggest it improves pain, diminishes ST segment changes, affects regional coronary blood flow and the analgesic effect is not prevented by naloxone.[29-33]

Spinal cord stimulation has been well described since its use in angina was described as a chance finding in a patient who had a stimulator for another reason in 1984.[34] Studies have confirmed improved quality of life, fewer ischaemic episodes and reduced frequency of hospital admissions.[35-38] Underlying myocardial ischaemia does not appear to be masked and mortality rates appear to be similar to those of the general population with ischaemic heart disease.

Patient selection is of paramount importance and the procedure (which usually requires general anaesthesia) carries risks of infection and haematoma formation. Many such patients are anticoagulated, which adds to the difficulty. However, when compared to coronary artery bypass graft (CABG) surgery, one study reported similar benefits, with reduction in frequency of angina attacks and use of short-acting nitrates, although surgery showed additional improvement in ischaemia on exercise testing six months postoperatively.[39] It has been suggested as a useful alternative to CABG surgery in high-risk patients.

Anorexia/cachexia, nausea, constipation, dry mouth

Anorexia is a troublesome issue. Again, a commonsense approach looking for reversible problems such as oral candidiasis, untreated nausea and ill-fitting dentures is important. Small meals, attractively presented, and avoidance of cooking smells if possible are often helpful, as is altering practice to 'grazing' smaller snacks during the day. Sometimes the issue of food intake can cause distressing conflict between carers and the patient. Because mealtimes are inherently part of our whole family/social structure, tensions can arise and patients feel under pressure to eat. A common approach of eating for enjoyment, little and often, may take the pressure off the patient. However, this will entail an honest discussion regarding the stage of disease, which many professionals find difficult. Sometimes patients are not eating enough because they do not have the energy to prepare themselves a meal, and the practical step of getting help in this regard may be all that is needed. However, before this supervenes it is important to pay attention to diet, as there is evidence that some patients with clinically stable heart failure are in negative calorie balance[40] – in this situation advice from a dietician may be beneficial. Weight loss that is clearly not due to diuresis is a poor sign, and may indicate that the anorexia is part of the cachexia syndrome of advanced heart failure. The syndrome is caused by inflammatory cytokines and leads to a catabolic/anabolic imbalance.[41] There is little evidence to suggest that increasing calorie intake *at this advanced stage* is likely to have benefit.

Patients can be nauseated due to drug side effects (aspirin, spironolactone, digoxin toxicity), gut wall or liver congestion, or renal failure. Constipation is common, due to reduced mobility, restricted fluid and food intake, or diuresis, and in itself can cause nausea. A prokinetic anti-emetic such as metoclopramide (10–20 mg tds) may help both situations, and is probably more reliably absorbed from the gut than domperidone. Domperidone does come in suppository form, which is occasionally useful if a patient is vomiting, wishes to stay at home and does not want a syringe driver for subcutaneous administration. A good alternative to metoclopramide would be low-dose haloperidol (0.5–3 mg) which can be used once daily at night. Anti-emetics with a strong anticholinergic action (such as cyclizine or hyoscine) should be avoided if possible, because of potential cardiac toxicity and exacerbation of constipation. Choice of laxative is also important. Many patients are fluid restricted, which can create problems with ispaghula husk. Softeners such as lactulose or polyethylene glycol, which may need augmenting with a stimulant such as senna, are better.

A dry mouth (xerostomia) may be due to drugs, particularly diuretics, analgesics and anti-emetics. Mucin-based saliva substitutes and using sugar-free chewing gum as a saliva stimulant may be helpful. Avoid acids in dentate patients, either in artificial saliva or as vitamin C or in fruit juices, since they cause demineralisation of teeth and other oral problems. Look for and treat oral candidiasis.

Skin care (cellulitis, dry/itchy skin, oedema)

Skin care is an overlooked problem. Chronic peripheral oedema can result in dry, thinned, friable skin at risk of cellulitis. Co-morbidities such as diabetes or peripheral vascular disease may also complicate the picture by causing poor peripheral circulation. In general, the patient's skin may become dry and itchy. Simple measures such as regular application of aqueous cream or similar moisturiser can help. The addition of menthol, as a cooling agent, to the cream can give further benefit. Sometimes itch may be present because of concomitant renal failure. Mirtazapine has been reported in case studies to help.[42] An open label trial of 4 mg twice daily ondansetron in 11 ambulatory patients on long-term peritoneal dialysis reported benefit in uraemic pruritus, but a cross-over placebo-controlled study did not show any statistically significant improvement.[43,44] Presumably any benefit is because serotonin is a chemical mediator in itch pathways. Thalidomide inhibits pro-inflammatory mediators, and has been described as helpful in uraemic itch when used in 29 dialysis patients with resistant itch.[45] Half the patients reported improvement with 100 mg at night. In the UK, there are stringent regulations governing the prescription of thalidomide, where both prescriber and patient have to be registered with the supplier (Pharmion) and drugs dispensed following informed written consent and telephone surveys completed each month by patient and doctor.

Conclusions

Physical symptom burden in heart failure is high. Historically, patients with heart failure have had patchy attention to symptom control and little access to supportive or specialist palliative care services. Access has been hampered by funding and resource issues, and compounded by a lack of robust evidence on effectiveness and cost-effectiveness of interventions. There is also a perception among some cardiologists and palliative care professionals that patients with heart failure would not feel comfortable in a hospice environment. Cardiologists may also find it difficult to know how to broach the subject of referral to palliative care, as it often involves discussion about prognosis, wishes regarding resuscitation attempts and other topics, which may be uncomfortable and difficult. Prognosis itself is notoriously difficult, and many cardiologists will put off this discussion until it is too late to involve palliative care services. It is hoped that the suggestions given in this chapter for possibilities for improvement in patients' symptom burden will encourage earlier use of palliative approaches. Many of the skills described in this chapter are within the scope of generic services. Heart failure nurse specialists are ideally placed to bridge the gap between the specialities (including primary care). As these posts are developed across the country, the hope is for a more seamless service for patients with heart failure so that it is no longer said 'you've got to have cancer to have good palliative care'.

References

1 Doyle D, Hanks G, Cherney N, Calman K (eds). *Oxford Textbook of Palliative Medicine* (3e). Oxford University Press, Oxford, 2004.

2 McCarthy M, Lay M, Addington-Hall J. Dying from heart disease. *J R Coll Physicians* 1996; **30**: 325–8.

3 Stanek EJ, Oates MB, McGhan WF *et al*. Preferences for treatment outcomes in patients with heart failure: symptoms versus survival. *J Cardiac Fail* 2000; **6**: 225–32.

4 Leidy NK, Rentz AM, Zycznski TM. Evaluating health-related quality-of-life outcomes in patients with congestive heart failure. A review of recent randomised controlled trials. *Pharmacoeconom* 1999; **15**: 19–46.

5 Anderson H, Ward C, Eardley A *et al*. The concerns of patients under palliative care and a heart failure clinic are not being met. *Pall Med* 2001; **15**: 279–86.

6 Murray SA, Boyd K, Kendall M *et al*. Dying of lung cancer or cardiac failure: prospective qualitative interview study of patients and their carers in the community. *BMJ* 2002; **325**: 929–32.

7 Gibbs JS, McCOy AS, Gibbs LM *et al*. Living with and dying from heart failure: the role of palliative care. *Heart* 2002; **88**(Suppl 2): ii, 36–9.

8 Luzier AB, DiTusa L. Underutilisation of ACE inhibitors in heart failure. *Pharmacotherapy* 1999; **19**: 1296–307.

9 Gheorghiade M, Gattis WA, O'Connor CM. Treatment gaps in the pharmacologic management of heart failure. *Rev Cardiovasc Med* 2002; **3**(Suppl 3): S11–19.

10 Moore S, Corner J, Haviland J *et al*. Nurse-led follow-up and conventional medical follow up in management of patients with lung cancer: randomised trial. *BMJ* 2002; **325**: 1145–52.

11 Fischer MD. Chronic heart failure and morphine treatment. [Letter; Comment] *Mayo Clin Proc* 1998; **73**: 194.

12 Cushen M. Palliative care in severe heart failure. *BMJ* 1994; **308**: 717.

13 Williams SG, Wright DJ, Diesch JP *et al*. Effect of low dose diamorphine on exercise capacity in patients with chronic heart failure. *Heart* 2001; **85**(Suppl 1): 4.

14 Chua TP, Harrington D, Ponikowski P *et al*. Effects of dihydrocodeine on chemosensivity and exercise tolerance in patients with chronic heart failure. *J Am Coll Cardiol* 1997; **29**: 147–52.

15 Timmis AD, Rothman MT, Henderson MA *et al*. Haemodynamic effects of intravenous morphine in patients with acute myocardial infarction complicated by severe left ventricular failure. *BMJ* 1980; **280**: 980–2.

16 Johnson MJ, McDonagh TA, Harkness A *et al*. Morphine for the relief of breathlessness in patients with chronic heart failure – a pilot study. *Eur J Heart Fail* 2002; **4**: 753–6.

17 Farncombe M, Chater S. Case studies outlining use of nebulised morphine for patients with end-stage chronic lung and cardiac disease. *J Pain Symptom Manage* 1993; **8**: 221–5.

18 Moore DP, Weston AR, Hughes JM *et al*. Effects of increased inspired oxygen concentrations on exercise performance in chronic heart failure. *Lancet* 1992; **339**: 850–3.

19 Restrick LJ, Davies SW, Noone L *et al*. Ambulatory oxygen in chronic heart failure. *Lancet* 1992; **340**: 1192–3.

20 Russell SD, Koshkarian GM, Medinger AE *et al*. Lack of effect of increased inspired oxygen concentrations on maximal exercise capacity or ventilation in stable heart failure. *Am J Cardiol* 1999; **84**: 1412–16.

21 Booth S, Wade R, Johnson MJ *et al*. The use of oxygen in the palliation of breathlessness. A report of the expert working group of the scientific committee of the association of palliative medicine. *Resp Med* 2004; **98**: 66–77.

22 Silverberg DS, Wexler D, Blum M *et al*. Effect of correction of anaemia with erythropoietin and intravenous iron in resistant heart failure in octogenarians. *Israel Medical Association Journal: Imaj* 2003; **5**: 337–9.

23 ExTraMATCH Collaborative. Exercise training meta-analysis of trials in patients with chronic heart failure (ExTraMATCH) *BMJ* 2004; **328**: 189–92.

24 Beniaminovitch A, Lang CC, LaManca J *et al*. Selective low-level leg muscle training alleviates dyspnoea in patients with heart failure *J Am Coll Cardiol* 2002; **40**: 1602–8.

25 McConnell TR, Mandak JS, Sykes JS *et al*. Exercise training for heart failure patients improves respiratory muscle endurance, exercise tolerance, breathlessness and quality of life. *J Cardiopulmon Rehab* 2003; **23**: 10–16.

26 World Health Organization. *Cancer Pain Relief* (2e). World Health Organization, Geneva, 1996, p.74.

27 Heerdink E, Leufkens H, Herings R *et al*. NSAIDs associated with increased risk of congestive heart failure in elderly patients taking diuretics. *Arch Intern Med* 1998; **158**: 1108–12.

28 Douglas CA, Moore RKG, Leach A *et al*. Modified-release opioids improve pain control and health-related quality of life in patients with complex cardiac chest pain. *Pall Med* 2004; **18**: 740–1.

29 Bueno EA, Mamtani R, Frishman WH. Alternative approaches to the medical management of angina pectoris: acupuncture, electrical nerve stimulation, and spinal cord stimulation. *Heart Dis* 2001; **3**: 236–41.

30 Borjesson M, Eriksson P, Dellborg M *et al*. Transcutaneous electrical nerve stimulation in unstable angina pectoris. *Coronary Artery Disease* 1997; **8**: 543–50.

31 Jessurun GA, Tio RA, De Jongste MJ *et al*. Coronary blood flow dynamics during transcutaneous electrical nerve stimulation for stable angina pectoris associated with severe narrowing of one major coronary. *Am J Cardiol* 1998; **82**: 921–6.

32 Mannheimer C, Emanuelsson H, Waagstein F. The effect of transcutaneous electrical nerve stimulation (TENS) on catecholamine metabolism during pacing-induced angina pectoris and the influence of naloxone. *Pain* 1990; **41**: 27–34.

33 West PD, Colquhoun DM. TENS in refractory angina pectoris. Three case reports. *Med J Austr* 1993; **158**: 488–9.

34 Sandric S, Meglio M, Bellocci F *et al*. Clinical and electro-cardiographic improvement of ischaemic heart disease after spinal cord stimulation. *Acta Neurochir* Suppl 1984; **33**: 543–6.

35 DeJongste MJL, Hautvast RWM, Hillege JL, Lie KI on behalf of the Working Group on Neurocardiology. Efficacy of spinal cord stimulation as adjuvant therapy for intractable angina pectoris. *J Am Coll Cardiol* 1994: **23**: 1592–7.

36 DeJongste MJL, Haaksma J Hautvast RWM *et al*. Effects of spinal cord stimulation on myocardial ischaemia during daily life in patients with severe coronary artery disease. A prospective ambulatory electrocardiographic study. *Br Heart J* 1994; **71**: 413–18.

37 Sanderson JE, Brooksby P, Waterhouse D *et al*. Epidural spinal electrical stimulation for severe angina: a study of its effect on symptoms, exercise tolerance, and degree of ischaemia. *Eur Heart J* 1992: **13**: 628–33.

38 Murray S, Carson KGS, Collins PD *et al*. Spinal cord stimulation significantly reduces hospital readmissions in patients with intractable angina pectoris. *Heart* 1998: **79** (Suppl): 48.

39 Mannheimer C, Eliasson T, Augustinsson L-E *et al*. Electrical stimulation versus coronary artery bypass surgery in severe angina pectoris. The ESBY study. *Circulation* 1998; **97**: 1157–63.

40 Pasini E, Opasich C, Pastoris O *et al*. Inadequate nutritional intake for daily life activity of clinically stable patients with chronic heart failure. *Am J Cardiol* 2004; **93**: 41A–43A.

41 Anker SD, Sharma R. The syndrome of cardiac cachexia. [Review] *Int J Cardiol* 2002; **85**: 51–66.

42 Davis MP, Frandsen JL, Walsh D *et al.* Mirtazepine for pruritus. *J Pain Symptom Manage* 2003; **25**: 288–91.

43 Balaskas EV, Bamihas GI, Karamouzis M *et al.* Histamine and serotonin in uraemic pruritus: effect of ondansetron in CAPD – pruritic patients. *Nephron* 1998; **78**: 395–402.

44 Murphy M, Reaich D, Pai P *et al.* A randomised, placebo-controlled, double-blind trial of ondansetron in renal itch. *Br J Dermatol* 2003; **148**: 314–17.

45 Silva SR, Viana PC, Lugon NV *et al.* Thalidomide for the treatment of uraemic pruritus; a cross over, randomised, double blind trial. *Nephron* 1994; **67**: 270–3.

Chapter 6

Supportive care: psychological, social and spiritual aspects

Scott Murray, Marilyn Kendall, Richard Lehman and Miriam Johnson

Patients with heart failure are affected in all aspects of their lives, and patients facing a life-limiting illness should receive attention to their spiritual and psychosocial needs, as well as the physical.[1] The physical symptoms and disabilities reach out and entangle the way they cope, their emotional buoyancy, their ability to work (and hence their finances), and their role in society and within their family. It spreads to their very meaning of life and affects their family and others caring for them. Conversely, social stability and supports, financial security, living accommodation and neighbourhood will affect coping and the ease with which help can be accessed. Supportive care is an essential part of management, but its importance has only recently been emphasised alongside that of medical care. In fact, the perception that the doctor has little or no role in anything other than medication can leave the practitioner feeling helpless and frustrated. A realisation that all healthcare professionals can recognise the multi-domain issues affecting their patients, deal with what they can and refer to appropriate other agencies or professionals as necessary would lead to such supportive care.

Supportive care is defined by the National Council for Palliative Care as care that:

> *... helps the patient and their family to cope with cancer and treatment of it – from pre-diagnosis, through the process of diagnosis and treatment, to cure, continuing illness or death and bereavement. It helps the patients to maximise the benefits of treatment and to live as well as possible with the effects of the disease. It is given equal priority alongside diagnosis and treatment.[2]*

The level and type of support that should be available for adults with cancer is detailed in the NICE guidelines.[3] A helpful adaptation of these with reference to patients suffering from heart failure has been produced by the Coronary Heart Disease Collaborative in the UK (recently renamed 'Heart Improvement Project').[4]

Until recently, most research studies and health service developments for people with heart failure focused on medication to reduce mortality and breathlessness, and interventions to prevent hospital readmissions. However, a number of recent studies have sought to gain an understanding of the lived experience of people with heart failure and their informal and professional carers, which can be used to inform the development of a broader range of services that are suitable, accessible and acceptable to patients and carers.[5–13] In a recent study in Edinburgh, 20 people with severe heart failure, and their carers, were interviewed at three-monthly intervals for up to one year.[6] These patients described a pattern of progressive decline, punctuated by episodes of acute deterioration and admission to hospital, growing dependence and an unpredictable terminal phase. Most had been given little information about their illness and prognosis, and gave graphic accounts of uncontrolled symptoms, poor quality of life, and emotional and spiritual distress. Their experience was compared with that of 20 patients dying with lung cancer (summarised in Box 6.1) and it was found that they often had very different needs and experiences, a contrast that serves to highlight many of the key issues and debates in the care of heart failure.

Box 6.1 Summary of the comparative research study[6]

Results: Heart failure patients had a different illness trajectory from the more linear and predictable course of lung cancer patients. In contrast to lung cancer patients, those with cardiac failure had little information about, and a poor understanding of, their condition and prognosis. They were less involved in decision making. Frustration, progressive losses, social isolation, and the stress of balancing and monitoring a complex medication regimen dominated the lives of cardiac failure patients. Heart patients received less health, social and palliative care services, and care was often poorly co-ordinated.

Conclusions: The experience of dying from these two common conditions was contrasting. Care for people with advanced progressive illnesses is currently prioritised by diagnosis rather than need. Patients, carers and professionals perceive the need to address this inequity. End-of-life care for patients with advanced cardiac failure should be proactive and designed to meet their specific needs.

Although most people talked about the physical aspects of their heart condition, and other illnesses, generally it was the wider aspects, the ways in which their illnesses had impacted upon their daily and social lives, and had compromised their ability to maintain their sense of self, that concerned them most. Many spoke of the 'impossible dream' of living the ordinary life that they used to take for granted, and felt they had been abandoned by the health and social care services.

Psychological problems

Psychological problems are common in chronic illness. Heart failure patients may struggle to cope with increasing debilities and shrinking abilities. Previous ways of coping may be helpful, but others less so. Patients may suffer adjustment reactions to progressive losses, which are in effect like sequential bereavements. While many patients work through these successfully, just as many people adjust to bereavement, others fail to adjust, and anxiety and depression may ensue.

Coping

Such is the resilience of human nature that the majority of patients cope with major health issues without help from healthcare professionals. Of those who do require assistance, probably only a few need the experience and training of clinical psychologists and psychiatrists – the majority managing with the skills of the general practitioner, heart failure nurse, cardiologist or palliative physician. It is, however, important to gain an understanding of how the patient usually copes (*see also* Chapter 7). Asking questions such as 'How would you describe yourself before you were ill?', 'What are your strengths?', 'How have you coped with hard times in the past?', can demonstrate coping strategies learned over many years, and are likely to be the ones used under stress. This assessment is also useful to remind the patient of the person they are, as this sense can be lost in one who has become overwhelmed by difficulties and ill health. Often during this process the patient will be able to suggest ways they can help themselves, thus taking back some control over the situation. This is important if there is to be a shared decision-making procedure for treatment. If not done, this may result in a decreasing spiral where the patient feels they are 'lost' in medical management they neither want nor understand, in the face of seemingly inevitable deteriorating physical condition. However, it is important to remember that patients do cope differently, and some do not wish, or are not able, to participate in such joint decision making. There is no mysterious technique needed to determine this – asking the patient usually suffices. 'What is your understanding of your condition?', 'Would you like to know more?', 'What do you think of the treatment plan so far?', 'Would you rather leave that decision to me, or would you like me to discuss it further?'

The way heart failure patients cope with their illness may be mirrored in how they approach understanding their drug treatment. In 2003, 37 patients with heart failure were interviewed and videotaped as part of the DIPEx project (www.dipex.org).[14] Looking at the heart failure interviews, it became clear that the patients fell into three broad categories.

- The first group seemed to show little understanding of their illness: despite agreeing to a study which mentioned 'heart failure' repeatedly and explicitly, half of them did not realise they had the condition. None of them knew what their drugs were intended to do, but did as they were told and left it at that.
- A second group showed greater awareness of their condition and understood part of their drug treatment, and those with access to specialist heart failure nurses found them to be 'a lifeline'. But when it came to changes of treatment, they felt that it was best to leave it to their doctors.
- The third (and smallest) group took an active interest in their condition and its treatment, and wanted to share in decision making.

Clearly some of these differences reflect the educational status of the patients. Some of the differences may also reflect the decision-making style, training and perceived role of the doctors who look after them, or patients' access to specialist nurses. However, this work demonstrates that patients vary widely in their capacity and their desire to be involved in the management of their illness.

A few years earlier, Stephen Buetow and his colleagues in Auckland, New Zealand, undertook similar interviews with 62 heart failure patients, specifically examining their coping strategies.[15] They found that the strategies used by patients to cope with their illness as a whole bear a close resemblance to the strategies we have just seen in relation to drug treatment.

- *Avoidance*: Such patients actively avoid information, especially if it is unfavourable.
- *Disavowal*: This appears to be a pre-conscious process. The patients understand the seriousness of the situation, but to reduce the resultant emotional strain they dissociate that awareness from its personal reality.
- *Acceptance*: Patients consciously accept the reality of their diagnosis, using understanding and control. Coping is through support from family and friends, drawing on humour and distracting activities.

In this large and representative sample of patients with heart failure, none displayed an outright refusal to acknowledge that anything was the matter with them. However, many patients used some kind of mechanism to downplay the seriousness of their condition, to avoid fear and despair, and to maintain hope. Any communication of diagnosis and prognosis, therefore, has to be done gently, realising that many will find this difficult, as it does not 'fit' with the way they are coping with their illness.

One of the advantages of a coping style that incorporates understanding and control is that it allows practical issues to be addressed with and for the patient. Unless a patient realises what is happening, it is difficult to arrange financial benefits, set up additional care or assess for living aids. Patients are denied the chance for end-of-life planning (legal and financial provision in the settling of affairs, personal choice for place of care) if they do not have a sufficient understanding. It is therefore imperative that communication is sensitive and skilful, particularly with patients who have less robust coping mechanisms. To do otherwise is to risk pushing a patient who is already struggling to maintain equanimity, into depression or anxiety. To avoid the situation by using euphemisms (*see* Chapter 7) is to potentially deny a patient their right to know and plan for the future.

Depression

Depression is a common condition in patients with heart failure, prevalence estimates ranging between 24% and 42%.[16] As with depression in patients with cancer, it often goes undiagnosed and untreated, and is considered 'understandable'. Similarly, it can be difficult to recognise, as many of the somatic symptoms are present due to the underlying physical illness.

Depression appears to be an important factor in heart failure, independently associated with repeat hospital admissions and a worse prognosis.[17–21] Heart failure has also been noted as a pre-morbid condition in a significant proportion of elderly patients who committed suicide.[22] Moreover, there is now evidence that depression in the general population is a risk factor for developing heart failure. Depression and heart failure share pathophysiological mechanisms and psychosocial issues. It is thought that augmentation of catecholamine release, pro-inflammatory cytokines[23] and platelet activation may be a mechanism whereby depression could make heart failure worse, or even cause it, perhaps by arrhythmias. Depression is also associated with poor social support, which in turn is associated with a poorer outcome in heart failure. Depression affects compliance with drug and exercise treatments; thus it is not surprising to find that one makes the other worse. A prospective study[24] of patients with heart failure showed that patients who lived alone, had a history of alcohol abuse, perceived their medical care to be an economic burden and were of poor health status (measured by Kansas City Cardiomyopathy Questionnaire) were more likely to develop depressive symptoms. Each factor was an independent predictor, but if three were present, then the incidence of developing depression increased to 69.2%.

Treatment with selective serotonin re-uptake inhibitors (SSRIs) seems to be helpful and safe.[25] Indeed there is evidence that their anti-platelet activity has an additional effect over and above aspirin.[26] Tricyclic antidepressants are best avoided because of their anticholinergic, and hence pro-arrhythmic activity,[25] and likewise, venlafaxine has been found to be associated with an increased risk of arrhythmias, although trazodone appears to be safe. Mirtazapine appears to be both safe and effective. Psychological treatments such as cognitive behavioural and stress management techniques seem to be helpful,[27] and there is some evidence that exercise programmes may also help mood.[28] It is yet to be seen whether treated depression still carries an adverse prognosis in heart failure.

Anxiety

In the general population, anxiety is often present with depression, and may be one of its presenting features. Anxiety can exacerbate the symptom of breathlessness, and superimposed panic attacks can be extremely distressing for patient and carer alike. However, although there is increasing evidence that depression carries a worse prognosis in heart failure, the literature (such as it is) is less clear for anxiety. Jiang *et al.* in a prospective study of 291 patients, found that although anxiety and depression were both highly correlated in heart failure patients, only depression carried a worse prognosis.[29] Some writers have concluded that greatly heightened anxiety is not a feature of chronic heart failure,[30] although they did acknowledge the paucity of the literature – and indeed, Jiang's work was not available at the time of that particular review. It has also been suggested that as natriuretic peptides show anxiolytic properties in rodent studies and patients with panic disorder, they may also protect against anxiety in heart failure.[31] Herrmann-Lingen *et al.* showed that the severity of chronic heart failure was significantly related to pro-atrial natriuretic peptide (pro-ANP) levels, poor physical quality of life, vital exhaustion and depression.[31] However they found no correlation between anxiety and severity of disease. Levels of pro-ANP were negatively correlated with anxiety. They suggested this might be part of a negative-feedback loop limiting psychological distress and subsequent adverse autonomic consequences in severe heart failure.

Experience tells us, however, that a level of anxiety – even if not often reaching anxiety state severity – is frequently found in patients with chronic disability, such as those with heart failure. Breathlessness, increasing restrictions and worries as to how they will 'manage' concern patients with heart failure. Dysfunctional breathing patterns may be partially alleviated with attention to anxiety management, and occasionally, judicious use of intermediate half-life benzodiazepines such as lorazepam or lormetazepam may be helpful. Awareness of unwanted effects is important and is discussed further in Chapter 5. Undisclosed anxieties and concerns may exacerbate the clinical situation, and good communication skills are important (*see* Chapter 7).

Uncertainty and hope

> '*I don't know how long I've got.' Mr K*

The course of heart failure, even in its advanced stages, involves a great deal of uncertainty. Uncertainty is generally seen in a negative way: in most life situations, it gives rise to anxiety, and we try to minimise it. However, there is a positive side to uncertainty as well, as Buetow *et al.*[15] point out. They urge general practitioners to 'befriend' uncertainty in life-threatening illness, because it leaves room for hope. Such hope is not illusory either, because many patients with heart failure do survive for long periods against the odds.

In the Edinburgh study,[6] all the participants spoke of having good days and bad days. However, all found it hard to predict when these would be, and consequently how to plan their lives. Although they wanted to be optimistic about their progress, this was hard to maintain in the face of continual setbacks.

> '*I try to carry on a normal life, but it seems to be one step forward and two back.' Mrs KK*

> '*I know I won't get better, but I hope it won't get any worse.' Mrs BB*

People struggled to maintain a normal life while swinging, often in the same day, from hope to despair. Consequently, people often gave parallel accounts of trying to remain positive while also facing the real possibility of dying.

Social problems

The practicalities of daily living can become insuperable problems. From the devastation of giving up work if not already retired, to maintaining housework, shopping, gardening, and the more personal issues of bathing and toileting. Financing paid help, if there are insufficient family and friends to help, or indeed the patient does not wish to put such a burden on those they love, can be hard. In the UK, there is some non-means-tested state assistance in disability living or attendance allowances, but these can be daunting to apply for, and if turned down, difficult to appeal against when up against demoralising bureaucracy, unless there is an advocate for the patient. Because of the difficulty of prognosis and communication, these allowances are often not claimed under a 'fast-track' system which would mean the money coming through while still timely. Other non-social security grants are available, but those patients who do not have a well-informed nurse specialist are often disadvantaged in both knowing about them and being able to decipher complicated applications.

The decision to go into nursing home care can be a deeply distressing one for many, but struggling to maintain independence in their own home can also be very frightening for those unable to cope. Access to the multiprofessional team such as physiotherapy and occupational therapy can be difficult in the community, where such resources may be relatively scarce. Funding can also be a problem with regard to what must be paid for by the patient and what will come from the health or social services budget. Where it is agreed that something, e.g. a stairlift, can be provided, it can take time to be fitted. This is often an area where referral to the specialist palliative care services reveals a hitherto unmet need.

There does appear to be a relationship between poor social support and hospital admissions and mortality.[32] Single marital status correlated with readmission and death in a prospective study of 257 patients.[33] Indeed, marital status on its own does not seem to be the whole story, and the *quality* of the relationship has an independent effect on mortality.[34]

Emotional and practical problems were immensely important for the interviewees in the Edinburgh study,[6] but they found it much more difficult to get help with these areas. Things like simply managing the activities of daily living – bathing, dressing, shopping, cooking, and cleaning, trying to continue meaningful social interactions by keeping up holidays, hobbies, and visits to family and friends, dealing with financial matters, and obtaining suitable housing and transport proved extremely difficult.

Most became experts in the logistics of their routine journeys, knowing the barriers such as hills they faced, where toilets were, and shops they could stop and pretend to look at. For some, the smallest household job required major planning. Over time, patients lost confidence, making it even less likely that they would go out.

> 'The tiniest incline is a mountain to me now.' Mrs LL

> 'I'm a home bird now. I like to be near… You feel safe when you're at home.' Mr T

> 'I would give the world to be able to go out now.' Mr K

As a consequence, people's ability to maintain satisfying roles and relationships diminished, and so their self-esteem declined and feelings of dependency grew. Low mood and anxiety were prevalent among both patients and carers as they struggled with the daily grind of living with heart failure.

> 'I can't do anything else … I feel like I'm in prison here with him. I can't go out and each day is just like the last.' Carer of Mr Z

A few were able to keep more cheerful, particularly if they had supportive family relationships or were able to hope that things would not get any worse. Humour, a determination not to be beaten, pragmatism and stoicism were all apparent, but often fragile coping strategies and feelings of uselessness or hopelessness were common.

Some patients said their quality of life was so poor that they would welcome death. These feelings were often not admitted to close family for fear of causing distress.

> 'Frustration – oh yes… I see her [his wife] doing things and it makes me feel guilty… I just can't do it… I find it very, very hard at times.' Mr K

> 'I think he probably needs a gun… if you were a horse, they would shoot you.' Carer of Mr N

Perceived ageism emerged, with many patients and carers feeling they had been written off. The frustration felt by general practitioners that little could be done for these patients, apart from changing the medication, was often conveyed to patients and carers.

> *'I want to be treated like a human being, not a lump of flesh everyone is trying to get rid of.' Mr E*

There was little evidence of support for informal carers. Partners and children often felt they had no choice about taking on the caring role and extra responsibilities in the changing relationship with their spouse or parent, a role that could continue for many years. Many carers seemed to see the reality of the situation, when patients wanted to maintain the pretence of managing well. People without an informal carer faced tremendous difficulties in trying to manage alone in the community.

People described a steadily shrinking social world, in which social isolation, co-morbidity and increasing disability were key issues. They spoke with regret of places they could no longer get to, people they could no longer see and hobbies they could no longer pursue. This shrinking world made it difficult for them to maintain any sense of having a meaningful life and worthwhile social interactions.

Clausen *et al.* comment on the Edinburgh study from a social worker's perspective.[35] They highlight six areas of concern from the patients' experience, in which social worker involvement could have made a difference:

- loss and dependency
- family-centred issues
- carers' needs
- practical tasks
- emotional and spiritual struggles
- support needs of staff.

There is little in the literature regarding the role of the social worker in meeting the needs of patients with anything other than cancer. The authors call to return to a holistic 'casework' model of social work rather than 'care management', which focuses only on specific 'identified needs' as a way of addressing some of these issues associated with chronic progressive ill health. They remind us that social workers can provide more than just practical aids and benefits, they can also be an advocate, support and counsellor.

Spiritual problems

Murray *et al.* demonstrated that spiritual issues were important, often the source of unmet need and inextricably linked with all the other problems.[6,36] Patients often looked back at their lives to try to make sense of why this illness had occurred. For some, this involved an element of guilt; one man with heart failure saying:

> *'Maybe this is God turning round and saying "I'm going to get you back"... because I've not always been a lily-white guy.' Mr HH*

Some struggled to find meaning in life, given the restrictions imposed by age, disability and a long-term condition. Often people were admitted to busy hospital wards, where spiritual and emotional needs went generally unrecognised:

> *'The staff are too busy, and you have to learn to look out for yourself. You just have to adapt. I try to hide my grief and be nice to others. That's what they want to see, someone coming in who's cheerful and doesn't complain.' Mr M*

Increasing disability altered people's self-image, and proposed solutions, such as using a wheelchair or having help with bathing, could be experienced as depersonalising and degrading, causing spiritual distress.

> *'She [the occupational therapist] decided I needed boards on the side of my bed, oh aye, that got me. So I said:"Are you going to leave me no dignity at all?" I never saw her again.' Mr E*

Topics that are recognised as markers of spiritual distress, such as difficult changes in relationships and social roles, increasing dependence on others for daily needs, feeling isolated and unsupported, lacking self-confidence, and feeling frustrated and depressed, formed major themes in the interviews. Some patients, attempting to vocalise feelings of spiritual distress, resisted being labelled as depressed.

> *'I'm not depressed… not really depressed… it's just a low feeling, and it's not a happy feeling, and you just never feel your life's worth anything at times.' Ms J*

Hope was difficult to maintain in such circumstances. Many patients spoke of feeling valueless and useless, nothing but a burden to others, and many expressed a wish for death.

> *'And I said, "I feel I can't go on." And yet, I don't have the courage, and I never could have the courage, to take my own life. I feel I've reached the end here. But I just wish somebody would come and put me out of my misery.' Mrs KK*

Many people spoke of the strength they drew from being able to maintain their relationships with their families. Opportunities to continue to give and receive love, to feel connected to their social world and to feel useful were highly valued.

> *'It's not wonderful but I can cope with it, I'm still at home, I'm with my family, I know that they still want me here and I can be of some help to them in looking after the grandchildren. It's a good enough life. It's still worth living, for me.' Mrs A*

Those people who were religious found comfort from the support of their church.

> *'And I get out to the church. My daughter comes every Sunday and takes me, because I can't walk there any more. All my life, even when I was in the army during the war, I would make every effort that I could to get there and that has always given me strength.' Mr K*

In the interviews, most general practitioners said they considered it their role to raise spiritual issues, but felt they lacked the time and training to carry out this role well. They tended to wait for cues from the patients, which were not always forthcoming, especially as patients were not at all sure if dealing with such issues was part of the general practitioner's role.

> *'But it's not possible with everyone. Some people are very open to it and others are like a brick wall… You can't make people talk to you about death and dying.' General practitioner of Mr V*

The spiritual needs of these heart failure patients, therefore, were characterised throughout by the hopelessness, loss of purpose, isolation and altered self-image associated with chronic illness and disability. These are common to most patients with advanced heart failure, whereas specifically religious issues are probably only significant for a minority.[37] For many people, spiritual needs are not expressed in the language of religion but in terms of the need to maintain a sense of self-worth, to have a useful role in life, retaining an active role with family and friends. The prospect of dying can lead to a deeper level of questioning and searching for meaning, and sometimes forgiveness, which can be a lonely struggle going on for months, hidden from health professionals and even from immediate family.

Health professionals may be wary of taking the initiative in exploring these issues, and indeed there is some evidence[37] that professionals can sometimes unwittingly contribute to some patients' feelings of worthlessness and loss of dignity. However, adequate time and sensitive use of listening skills, such as empathy and open questioning, can create conditions where patients and carers feel able to discuss their hopes and fears if they wish. It has recently been suggested that the ideal opening question might be 'Are you at peace?'.[38] When given the opportunity to discuss spiritual needs with professionals, some patients and carers in the Edinburgh study valued this greatly, both because it validated their concerns and because they felt cherished. Those most closely involved in looking after patients with advanced heart failure need therefore to be aware of the possibility of spiritual distress, and if they do not feel able to address it themselves, need to be able to access help from other sources, possibly including an experienced chaplain or counsellor.[39,40]

Death and dying

Although many had experienced 'brushes with death' during acute episodes, few patients had discussed their preferred place of death or wishes for end-of-life care with professionals. Most thought about dying in the context of ageing. Many had made plans with relatives for their funerals, and arrangements about money and property. The uncertainty of the prognosis made it difficult for patients and carers to know how imminent death would be, although there was awareness of being 'really ill'.

> 'Sometimes I'm afraid in the morning to go in... he's fading away before my eyes... It could be another year or two or it could be another week or two, it could be tomorrow. I don't know.' Carer of Mr N

A final admission to hospital was as likely to be due to a non-cardiac condition or increasing care needs beyond the capacity of informal carers and community services to cope. Once admitted, insensitive communication could cause distress.

> 'They just told us they had a plan... they said, we have a plan that if she arrests we will not be resuscitating her. Just as if it was nothing... it was terrible.' Daughter of Mrs P

Most people reflected on their poor present quality of life.

'I was sitting in a chair all night… I would be screaming for air… very, very fright-ening… I suppose it's like drowning really.' Mrs A

'It's a life but it's not much of a life. I'm ready for the knacker's yard.' Mrs P

Professionals perceived that there was much less support in the community, and fewer opportunities than for patients with cancer to die at home.

A system failure

Heart failure patients have huge problems in many areas of their life. At present, many of these would appear to be unheard and unmet by the current system. Healthcare professionals often do not register these issues, and assistance from the multiprofessional teams may be lacking. These themes were clearly seen in the Scottish study. Heart failure patients often described negative experiences of hospital admission, with poorly co-ordinated hospital care, and failure to recog-nise the involvement and expertise of carers. Seeing different doctors at each hospital appointment caused particular dissatisfaction. Lack of privacy and dig-nity, with noisy and hectic wards, allowed little time for personalised care.

Primary care contacts were mainly with the general practitioner. There was little planned community support. A few people had developed a long-term relationship with a key professional: a consultant, general practitioner or special-ist cardiac nurse. Taking an interest, caring about the person and good communication skills were valued. Specialist palliative care services were not generally involved and only a minority had access to a specialist cardiac nurse. Social services, financial benefits advice, carer support and respite were largely absent, and information and support from cardiac charities were little used. Care was based on a treatment-focused, medical model. Lack of services, failure to address end-of-life issues and episodes of acute deterioration meant these patients were less likely to die at home.

'I'm expecting it to be something catastrophic so planning and discussing it isn't really an issue.' General practitioner of Mrs F

General practitioners recognised that there were more resources for cancer pa-tients and felt frustrated by their own role, which seemed limited to monitoring and adjusting medication.

Conclusion

There is an urgent need for the key role of supportive care to be recognised and addressed. This should not wait until the situation is so complex that specialist palliative care is involved – rather, cardiology and primary care services should work together to elucidate and tackle the problems. Referral to appropriate agencies and benefits should be routine and done in advance. This could avoid emergency hospital admissions due to carer exhaustion and breakdown of the social situation. Clear communication and such advanced planning may also enable the patient to have true choice with regard to preferred place of death, rather than mere rhetoric.

References

1　Basta LL. End-of-life medical treatment of older cardiac patients. *Am J Ger Cardiol* 2004; **13**: 313–15.

2　NCPC definitions of supportive and palliative care. Briefing paper 11. London, National Council for Palliative Care, September 2002.

3　Improving supportive and palliative care for adults with cancer (www.NICE.org.uk), 2004.

4　Department of Health. Coronary Heart Disease Collaborative. Available from www.modern.nhs.uk/chd

5　Anderson H, Ward C, Eardley A *et al*. The concerns of patients under palliative care and a heart failure clinic are not being met. *Pall Med* 2001; **15**: 279–86.

6　Murray SA, Boyd K, Kendall M *et al*. Dying of lung cancer or cardiac failure: prospective qualitative interview study of patients and their carers in the community. *BMJ* 2002; **325**: 929–32.

7　Gibbs JS, McCoy AS, Gibbs LM *et al*. Living with and dying from heart failure: the role of palliative care. *Heart* 2002; **88**(Suppl 2): ii, 36–9.

8　National Council for Hospices and Specialist Palliative Care Services and Scottish Partnership Agency. *Reaching Out: specialist palliative care for adults with non-malignant diseases*. National Council for Hospices and Specialist Palliative Care Services and Scottish Partnership Agency, London, 1998.

9　Addington-Hall J, McCarthy M. Regional study of care of the dying: methods and sample characteristics. *Pall Med* 1995; **9**: 27–35.

10　Rideout E, Montemuro M. Hope, morale and adaptation in patients with chronic heart failure. *J Adv Nursing* 1986; **11**: 429–38.

11　Rogers AE, Addington-Hall JM, Abery AJ *et al*. Knowledge and communication difficulties for patients with chronic heart failure: qualitative study. *BMJ* 2000; **321**: 605–7.

12　McCarthy M, Addington-Hall J, Ley M. Communication and choice in dying from heart disease. *J Roy Soc Med* 1997; **90**: 128–31.

13　Hanratty B, Hibbert D, Mair F *et al*. Doctors' perceptions of palliative care for heart failure – a focus study. *BMJ* 2002; **325**: 581–5.

14　Field K, Ziebland S, McPherson A, Lehman R. 'Can I come off the tablets now?' A qualitative analysis of heart failure patients' understanding of their medication. *Family Practice* 2006 (in press).

15　Buetow S, Goodyear-Smith F, Coster G. Coping strategies in the self-management of chronic heart failure. *Fam Pract* 2001; **18**: 117–22.

16　Guck TP, Elsasser GN, Kavan MG *et al*. Depression and congestive heart failure. [Review] *Congestive Heart Failure* 2003; **9**(3): 163–9.

17　Joynt KE, Whellan DJ, O'Connor CM. Why is depression bad for the failing heart? A review of the mechanistic relationship between depression and heart failure. *J Cardiac Fail* 2004; **10**: 258–71.

18　Pasic J, Levy WC, Sullivan MD. Cytokines in depression and heart failure. *Pychosomat Med* 2003; **65**: 181–93.

19　De Denus S, Spinler SA, Jessup M *et al*. History of depression as a predictor of adverse outcomes in patients hospitalised for decompensated heart failure. *Pharmacother* 2004; **24**: 1306–10.

20　Murberg TA, Bru E, Svebak S *et al*. Depressed mood and subjective health symptoms as predictors of mortality in patients with congestive heart failure: a two-years follow up study. *Int J Psychiat Med* 1999; **29**: 311–26.

21　Junger J, Schellberg D, Muller-Tasch T *et al*. Depression increasingly predicts mortality in the course of congestive heart failure. *Eur J Heart Fail* 2005; **7**: 261–7.

22　Juurlink DN, Herrmann N, Szalai JP *et al*. Medical illness and the risk of suicide in the elderly. *Arch Intern Med* 2004; **164**: 1179–84.

23　Parissis JT, Adamopoulos S, Rigas A *et al*. Comparison of circulating proinflammatory cytokines and soluble apoptosis mediators in patients with chronic heart failure with versus without symptoms of depression. *Am J Cardiol* 2004; **94**: 1326–8.

24 Havranek EP, Spertus JA, Masoudi FA *et al.* Predictors of the onset of depressive symptoms in patients with heart failure. *J Am Coll Cardiol* 2004; **44**: 2333–8.

25 Alvarez Jr W, Pickworth KK. Safety of anti-depressant drugs in the patient with cardiac disease: a review of the literature. *Pharmacother* 2003; **23**: 754–71.

26 Serebruany VL, Glassman AH, Malinin AI *et al.* Selective serotonin reuptake inhibitors yield additional antiplatelet protection in patients with congestive heart failure treated with antecedent aspirin. *Eur J Heart Fail* 2003; **5**: 517–21.

27 Luskin F, Reitz M, Newll K *et al.* A controlled pilot study of stress management training of elderly patients with congestive heart failure. *Prev Cardiol* 2002; **5**: 168–72.

28 Koukouvou G, Kouidi E, Iacovides A *et al.* Quality of life, psychological and physiological changes following exercise training in patients with chronic heart failure. *J Rehab Med* 2004; **36**: 36–41.

29 Jiang W, Kuchibhatila M, Cuffe MS *et al.* Prognostic value of anxiety and depression in patients with chronic heart failure. *Circulation* 2004; **110**: 3452–6.

30 MacMahon KM, Lip GY. Psychological factors in heart failure: a review of the literature. *Arch Intern Med* 2002; **162**: 509–16.

31 Herrmann-Lingen C, Binder L, Klinge M *et al.* High plasma level of N-terminal pro-atrial natriuretic peptide associated with low anxiety in severe heart failure. *Psychosom Med* 2003; **65**: 517–22.

32 Luttik ML, Jaarsma T, Moser D *et al.* The importance and impact of social support on outcomes in patients with heart failure: an overview of the literature. *J Cardiovasc Nurs* 2005; **20**: 162–9.

33 Chin MH, Goldman L. Correlates of early hospital readmission or death in patients with congestive heart failure. *Am J Cardiol* 1997; **79**: 1640–4.

34 Coyne JC, Rohrbaugh MJ, Shoham V *et al.* Prognostic importance of marital quality for survival of congestive cardiac failure. *Am J Cardiol* 2001; **88**: 526–9.

35 Clausen H, Kendall M, Murray S *et al.* Would palliative care patients benefit from social workers' retaining the traditional 'casework' role rather than working as care managers? A prospective serial qualitative interview study. *Br J Soc Work* 2004; **35**: 1–9.

36 Murray SA, Kendall M, Boyd K *et al.* Exploring the spiritual needs of people dying of lung cancer or heart failure: a prospective qualitative interview study of patients and their carers. *Pall Med* 2004; **18**: 39–45.

37 Fitchett G, Murphy PE, Kim J *et al.* Religious struggle: prevalence, correlates and mental health risks in diabetic, congestive heart failure, and oncology patients. *Int J Psychiatry Med* 2004; **34**: 179–96.

38 Steinhauser KE, Voils CI, Glipp EC *et al.* 'Are you at peace?': one item to probe spiritual concerns at the end of life. *Arch Intern Med* 2006; **166**: 101–5.

39 Westlake C, Dracup K. Role of spirituality in adjustment of patients with advanced heart failure. *Prog Cardiovasc Nurs* 2001; **16**: 119–25.

40 Oates L. Providing spiritual care in end-stage heart failure. *Int J Palliat Nurs* 2004; **10**: 485–90.

Chapter 7

Communication in heart failure

Iain Lawrie and Suzanne Kite

> *Communication is often defined as to impart or make known, but its Latin derivation is helpful in emphasizing the sharing of information; communis means in common.*
> Dias *et al.*[1]

Heart failure is affecting more people, and affecting them for longer. Medical technology and therapeutics grow apace, and while 'cures' are few and far between, there are an expanding number of treatment options available. While mortality rates from heart failure have fallen[2,3] morbidity rates, due to the growing elderly population, may continue to rise.[2] Thus, there are more and more conversations to be had between doctors and patients, discussing the nature and course of heart failure, prognosis, treatment options, and patient preferences for end-of-life care. As with other medical developments, the ethics and communication skills necessary to permit partnerships with patients have lagged behind the demographics and technology. Very few patients with heart disease have been given the opportunity to discuss end-of-life issues despite the fact that many have recognised death to be imminent.[4,5] There is also evidence that people with heart failure have less understanding of their illness than in other chronic diseases,[6] perhaps because the term 'heart failure' may not be familiar to patients,[5] and consideration of imminent death is largely confined to exacerbations.[7] Many patients with heart failure are ready for, and would welcome, information regarding prognosis.[8] This would suggest that there is an unmet need in this area of care and also that there is room for improvement in how we communicate with patients with heart failure.

Great strides have been made in communication within oncology through research and dialogue with public, patients and professionals, and there is every reason to hope that the same will be true for heart failure. The need for enhanced communication has been recognised in recent policy documents[9] and there is a growing body of work in the healthcare literature.

The term 'communication' encompasses a number of processes and skills. There is a spectrum from the imparting of information at one end, to joint decision making in complex situations of uncertainty and subtle balancing of benefits, burdens and risks at the other. Active listening, the ability to elicit patient concerns and to tailor the *sharing* of information and collaborative partnership in decision making to individual patients are all skills which are necessary and can be learned. *How* we communicate is also as important as what we actually say.

Good communication can lead to identifiable benefits for patients, professionals and healthcare systems. Patients are given the opportunity to take a more active role in the management of their illness through being better informed and being included in decision making. This can have a positive effect on patients[10] and can lead to enhanced patient and carer satisfaction with care. Healthcare staff benefit, as improved communication with patients contributes to a more open relationship where responsibilities and decisions are shared. This can lead to improved clinical care and professional wellbeing.[11] Better-informed patients who are more involved in their own care have also been shown to have improved compliance with treatment regimens which, in turn, results in decreased rates of readmission to hospital.[12,13] Such effects have positive ramifications for both health professionals and the healthcare system. Conversely, lack of open communication can lead to a substandard level of care.[14]

In this chapter, we present an overview of communication in heart failure. We will examine what patients need and wish to know, and explore some of the potential barriers to effective communication for this patient group. We then review various strategies that have been tried in order to improve communication with heart failure patients and reflect on their effectiveness. Learning points that may be transferred from experience in oncology and palliative care will be considered, along with suggestions for how effective communication skills can be learned. Finally, ways forward for communication in specific situations common in heart failure care will be explored.

What might need to be communicated?

Heart failure is a complex diagnosis. Many aspects require patient involvement and further discussion. Explanation about the nature of the condition, what may have caused it, the physical changes that have occurred and the symptoms such changes might bring about all form part of the communication process. Discussion of symptoms leads to exploration of the effects and limitations such symptoms may have on their lives. Patients may want to know what management strategies are available, including both pharmacological and non-drug therapies, and potential burdens or side effects of treatment. This is especially true for cardiac transplantation. Discussion of prognosis is important so that patients and their families can make plans, but in a way that preserves hope, where possible. However, patients may not ask about prognosis unprompted. End-of-life care planning also involves discussion of more difficult topics such as changing emphasis of treatment, starting or stopping treatment including implantable cardioverter defibrillators (ICDs), future care planning, resuscitation status, and 'do-not-resuscitate' (DNR) orders and advance directives. All these topics are difficult for both patient and professional to discuss and require sensitivity in communication.

What do we know about what patients want?

I think the best physician is the one who has the providence to tell to the patients according to his knowledge the present situation, what has happened before, and what is going to happen in the future.
Hippocrates (470–410 BC)[15]

Often, there can be a chasm between what professionals *think* their patients want to know and what patients and their carers *actually* want to know, or not know. It is clear, however, that many patients and their carers wish for more information than professionals estimate.[16] In a study by Formiga et al.,[17] 64% of patients were aware of the chronic and progressive nature of their condition, but McCarthy and Addington-Hall reported that nearly half of patients in their study had been unable to get all the information they wanted.[18]

Nurses involved in the care of patients with heart failure have reported that professionals tend to focus the care they provide for this group of patients on symptom control and drug management.[19] However, patients and carers want a more holistic approach to their care, addressing information needs and psycho-social concerns,[20] as well as the physical aspects of their illness.

Much of the literature suggests that patients want open and honest discussions with the professionals involved in their care,[21] these discussions covering all aspects of their illness, both positive and negative. They want information and support on how to achieve a good quality of life during their illness,[22] and education regarding their medication and treatment.

Cardiopulmonary resuscitation is an issue that patients may have considered and wish to talk about. However, it may not be discussed, even in conversations around future care planning and advance directives.[23] Professionals should approach discussion of resuscitation in order to determine to what extent the patient wishes to be involved in making such decisions.[24]

Communication regarding prognosis can be difficult and many patients with advanced disease can be overly optimistic about their prognosis.[25,26] In one study, many more professionals than patients or carers believed that discussions regarding prognosis had already taken place,[27] suggesting that communication had not been effective. Such discussions are important to patients, particularly as their illness progresses and they have a limited time left to live.[27]

However, not all patients want frank and open discussion and this wish should be respected. Some are not open to receiving specific prognostic information, preferring to avoid receiving bad news.[28,29] This is demonstrated by a study which found that 100% of patients wanted the professionals caring for them to be honest but, at the same time, 91% also wanted them to maintain hope or be optimistic.[28]

> *Patients with disabling, progressive illnesses expect active care, but they also seek comfort, control and dignity.*
> Murray et al.[30]

Potential barriers to communication

> *…communication is only effective when the patient understands what the clinician has said.*
> Fried et al.[27]

Effective communication goes beyond *what* is said and what is done during an encounter with a patient. A great many factors can have a detrimental effect on the quality of the experience and its effectiveness. Such factors are often referred to as *barriers* to communication and can be described across a number of domains: patient, disease, professional and system.

Patient-related factors

There are a number of potential barriers to communication in patients with heart failure. Limited exercise tolerance, fatigue, breathlessness and medical co-morbidities are all prevalent in this patient group and can seriously restrict the patient's ability to both attend and actively participate in outpatient appointments.[8] Breathlessness and fatigue limit the patient's ability to tell their story, express their concerns and ask questions. Patients with heart failure tend to be older and co-morbid conditions, such as dementia, poor eyesight and hearing difficulties, are all more common in this group.[31]

Psychosocial functioning is often impaired in patients with heart failure,[32,33] and is described more fully in Chapter 6. Depression can impair decision making for a number of reasons, from the forming of negative inferences, to the reduced ability to think clearly, logically and constructively in complex situations. A high incidence of major depression (17–26%) has been reported among people with chronic heart failure.[34,35] Minor depression is also common, being present in almost a third of patients.[35] Increased mortality among patients with heart failure who are depressed has been documented.[34–37] Patients with heart failure with significantly altered mood also tend to display reduced compliance with disease management,[38–40] to consult their doctor more often and to have more frequent readmissions to hospital.[35] Depression can persist or worsen following hospital discharge.[34,41,42] Several characteristics of depressed mood (e.g. fatigue, inability to concentrate, hopelessness, lack of social interaction, paucity of speech) serve to confound the communication process and decrease the involvement of the patient in their care. Such symptoms, common in heart failure, may mask depression, and good communication skills are required both to diagnose and to manage depression.

The lack of a common language used by patients, carers and professionals is in itself a barrier to effective communication. All must be able to understand not only what is said, but also the associated meanings. As mentioned, the term 'heart failure' is often not used by patients.[5] This may be because it conjures up images of a part of their body that is gradually weakening, which they find difficult to cope with. The term itself can be very emotive; one 'fails' an exam or is in a marriage which fails, for example. Also, the term 'heart' is central to our sense of self, our seat of emotion, our being and life itself. It is, therefore, understandable that patients can avoid using the label of 'heart failure', and professionals need to be aware of this when discussing diagnosis. Alternatively, avoidance of the term may reflect the fact that they have not received sufficient information or explanation to understand their illness properly.

Patients may also attribute a lack of information and discussion to a reluctance by the professional to give them too much or inappropriate information.[8] Cues from the patient may also be subtle or missing. Patients attending outpatient clinics, for example, may prioritise the information they pass on to the professional, as they realise that such visits are often limited by time and the professional agenda is one of 'balancing and monitoring' medication and physical symptoms. Patients may not volunteer information or opinion, feeling that to express their own views or wishes may in some way seem ungracious. They may feel that the cardiologist has put so much effort into caring for them and they don't know how to say that they don't want a particular treatment.

This unconscious negotiation, whereby the patient tacitly accepts the professional agenda, can lead to a less than ideal exchange of information.

Disease-related factors

Other symptoms associated with cardiac insufficiency also affect communication. Confusion and poor short-term memory can have a significant impact on the ability to communicate effectively with friends, carers and professionals.[8] Patients with heart failure may have difficulty in retaining information,[43] which inhibits the process of building on previous encounters, developing discussions and assimilating information into a coherent overview of their disease, treatment and prognosis. This in turn makes discussion about patients' wishes about future care more difficult and can be a barrier to informed decision making.

The very variable and unpredictable course of the disease also poses significant challenges. The relapsing–remitting nature of heart failure means that professionals often find it difficult to identify appropriate stages at which to discuss certain management options or approach changes to the direction of care or prognosis. The possibility of death, especially sudden death, is often not discussed openly. In New York Heart Association (NYHA) class II heart failure, annual mortality is estimated at 5–15%, but 50–80% of these patients can die suddenly.[44–46] At later stages of the disease (NYHA class IV), the annual mortality is 30–70%, yet only 5–30% die suddenly.[47] Although these data may help to focus information more accurately in this difficult patient group, individuals often do not relate their situation to statistics and can interpret statistics in a number of ways.

Professional-related factors

Professionals cannot agree on a single definition of heart failure and, as a result, can be reluctant to use the term[5] or find it very difficult to explain the diagnosis to the patient. It can be particularly difficult to translate extensive knowledge about such a complex pathophysiological process into language appropriate for individual patients, and doctors may feel that the term 'heart failure' may reflect a higher degree of risk than they wish to convey.[48] Doctors can also believe that patients expect too much certainty, particularly with prognosis[49,50] and, being unable to provide this, can avoid communicating key information entirely. The disease is progressive and the course unpredictable, and professionals, through the inevitable inability to foresee deteriorations in their patients' illness trajectories, can feel impotent.

The professional may also see their role as one solely of monitoring medical treatment and may feel uncomfortable about extending the relationship into a more equal one of sharing of information and decision making. This may be a result of the 'traditional' model of undergraduate training in history taking and examination, where the focus has been on making a diagnosis and formulating a treatment plan. Recently, this approach has been questioned and has resulted in the development of the extended Calgary–Cambridge model,[51,52] which outlines and structures the skills that have been shown by research and theory to aid doctor–patient communication. In this model, history taking and examination is wholly integrated with forming a relationship with the patient in order that joint decision making can occur. Although relatively well developed in primary care, it is now beginning to form the basis of consultation skills training in some medical schools.[53] It is encouraging that future professionals may not only consider communication to be their job, but also that *how* they discuss the problem with the patient is of equal importance to the medical or surgical management of that problem. The past two decades have seen a marked change in the doctor–patient relationship, with paternalism largely replaced by a number of models where respect for patient autonomy is central.[54] Two of the main models are the 'client–provider' and the 'partnership' models. The former is more appropriate for well patients seeking specific procedures; the role of the doctor is technician and the patient is the decision-making client. The partnership model recognises the unique skills and perspectives of both patient and physician working together towards optimal care for the individual, and does require significant investment in time and understanding by the patient. Not all frail palliative care patients can meet the demands of the partnership model at all times and, in these situations, best interest considerations will help the doctor make decisions for the patient based on their known preferences and goals.[55] The range of coexisting models of the doctor–patient relationship raises the possibility of misunderstanding between any particular patient and their doctor regarding which model is desired and which is in operation. Establishing mutual expectations is an important element of good communication.

Health professionals have their own attitudes and emotions to contend with. Peter Kaye's work[56] in the field of breaking bad news can be generalised more widely in clinical practice. He describes how doctors can experience feelings of incompetence, embarrassment and of being 'powerless' and 'failing' the patient, as well as being reminded of their human vulnerability. They may feel awkward about showing emotion or sympathy, seen by some as anathema to their 'clinical' role. They may fear being blamed by patients or carers for the progression of the patient's illness and feel powerless in not being able to offer 'ready' cures. Some may fear unleashing an emotional reaction from the patient or their carers, which they will find hard to manage, or fear that distress itself may further harm the patient. Professionals can prefer to 'shield' the patient from bad news, perhaps in an attempt to prevent causing distress or damaging hope.[30,48] If an earlier patient consultation has not occurred as the professional would have liked, or has been awkward, subsequent interactions with other patients may be negatively affected.[57] All these emotions and thoughts, engendered in the professional in what can be stressful situations,[58,59] can inhibit open communication between patient and professional.

The reality is that heart failure is associated with very debilitating symptoms, social problems and suffering. Professionals try to balance providing patients with information with a desire to maintain their hope[60] in a condition where the limitations and burdens of disease are high and the prognosis is far from certain.

System-related factors

The 'mechanics' of the healthcare system also influence quality of communication for patients and carers. Care of patients with heart failure has been described as unco-ordinated,[61] with lack of continuity of care and community support contributing to repeated admissions and discharges between hospital and community sectors. When patients are admitted to hospital, they are not necessarily

Table 7.1 Barriers to communication

Barriers to communication	
Patient and disease-related factors	• Difficulty in attending and participating in clinic appointments due to symptoms • Co-morbidities such as dementia, poor eyesight and hearing • Depression • Lack of 'common language' • Tacit acceptance of professional agenda • Cognitive impairment • Relapsing–remitting nature of disease • Difficulty with prognosis
Professional-related factors	• No agreed single definition of the disease • Perception that patients want prognostic certainty • See role solely as monitoring medical treatment • Don't want to upset patients • Feeling of powerlessness
System-related factors	• Poorly co-ordinated care especially between primary and secondary care • Lack of planning and continuity of care • Time constraints

looked after by the same team of professionals as previously and medical records can be missing or their receipt delayed.

An absence of coherent, planned care of patients in the community, especially for those in the terminal stages of their disease, coupled with a lack of specialist support for general practitioners, represents a barrier to communication on a wider scale:

> '…because the consultants are managing patients when they're on the wards and the general practitioners are trying to manage them at home, they're falling between two stools, and that seems to me to be a real problem.'
> Cardiologist, in Hanratty et al.[61]

Both patients and professionals have identified that time constraints limit communication opportunities.[56] If time is too limited, patients' ideas, concerns and expectations cannot be fully explored and patients may be reluctant to 'bother the busy doctor'. Busy cardiology clinics, where 10-minute appointments are allocated, are not appropriate for the cardiologist to deal with the complexities of heart failure. Attention to the set-up and running of clinics, with increasing use of heart failure nurse specialists and facilities where discussions may be held in private, are helpful strategies. Table 7.1 summarises the potential barriers to communication.

Lessons learned in communication from other areas of medicine

Much of the work in communication in hospital medicine and healthcare over the past 40 years has been in the field of oncology. Forty years ago, cancer patients in the UK were rarely informed of their prognosis and had little opportunity to be involved in decision making regarding their management.[62] On the grounds that treatment options were limited and the prognosis even with such treatment was poor, it was considered cruel to burden patients with this information. However, pioneering oncologists and palliative care physicians realised that, far from reducing suffering, this approach added to patient and carer distress and isolation, and over the past 30 years doctors have become increasingly likely to give patients more information about their physical health.[63–65]

Early work in communication looked at how best to break bad news. Simple, step-by-step approaches were developed and communications skills teaching is now a core component of most undergraduate medical curricula and many training programmes for other health professionals. Indeed, the central role of good communication in the provision of effective healthcare has been recognised at a national level, such skills training being recognised in policy documents.[66]

Breaking bad news is just one aspect of communication in cancer care. Skills are also required in communication of prognosis, giving complex information, obtaining informed consent, discussions with relatives, eliciting and managing psychosocial concerns, and coping with the emotions of both patients and carers.

More recently, communication literature has addressed the area of communication and management of risk and uncertainty, not just in oncology, but in many areas of medicine. A growing body of work exists regarding how patients make health decisions and what they need, want and expect from health professionals. There is a move away from patients being seen as passive recipients of information towards a new role as informed and involved partners in shared decision making.

Key messages arising from the work in oncology can be generalised to other fields. The importance of telling patients the truth at a pace, and to a level, tailored to their individual needs is well established. Such information is necessary for patients to make informed choices about treatment, their personal lives, and how and where they spend their time. Informing patients sensitively, empathetically and honestly respects their autonomy and helps to build the trusting professional relationships necessary at a time of crisis. Conversely, withholding information tends to compound fear and anxiety while removing the basis of trust, leaving patients scared and isolated. The vast majority of patients want to be well informed, but not all do. A significant minority would prefer to leave 'bad news' for now and face the consequences later, and it usually transpires that this is an enduring, lifelong coping strategy which may have served them well. Such situations require even greater sensitivity in negotiating the pace and timing at which information is shared. It should not be assumed that professionals 'instinctively' know how much information and how great a role in decision making individual patients want at any particular time. Preferences can and do fluctuate over time. It is important for professionals to question their assumptions, particularly if they are making generalisations based on gender, age, culture or educational background, as these are unreliable predictors. On the whole, younger patients want more information and to be more involved in decision making,[67] but so may certain older individuals. An individual approach is needed and the best approach is to talk with the patient.

However, such skills in sensitive and empathic communication and negotiation require training and support. The day-to-day barriers of time pressures and lack of privacy, combined with the emotionally demanding nature of the work, can erode good practice in even the most skilled. End-of-life discussions challenge us all, exposing our own beliefs and fears about death and dying. Addressing end-of-life concerns in others may be very discomforting. Communication skills training offers the opportunity to step back and to confront one's own professional and personal insecurities while learning a structured approach to communication, and has been shown to lead to improved attitudes, confidence and skills in participants.[68–70]

Oncologists and palliative care specialists have learned to reflect on the language they use in order to avoid ambiguity. Terms such as 'bladder warts', 'growths', 'tumours', 'cure of local disease', 'progressing' and even 'mischief' have all, for example, been found to be misleading (deliberately or otherwise) and are best avoided.

Step-by-step models of sharing bad news have been developed.[56,71] Such models emphasise the need to pace discussions, in order that difficult information can be conveyed with the patient feeling that they have some control over the direction of the conversation and are not overwhelmed. Preparatory steps include finding a suitable location which affords some privacy and freedom from interruptions, ensuring that appropriate people are present, especially a friend or family member if the patient wishes, having necessary notes and investigation results available, and clarifying the purpose of the discussion and the patient's understanding of what has led up to this point. Such preparation often affords the patient a 'warning shot' of what is to come and, as the doctor starts to deliver the news, more signals may be given to enable the patient to centre themselves. An example might be:

Doctor: *Your GP asked you to come to clinic because your symptoms were causing concern. Your recent tests have shown why you have been feeling so tired. Would you like me to explain the results?*

Patient nods.

Doctor: *I'm afraid to say that it is serious…*

Patient looks away… doctor pauses…

Doctor: *Would you like me to go on?*

Patient: *I've got cancer haven't I?*

Doctor: *I'm sorry to say that, yes, the results did show cancer.*

This brief excerpt illustrates the use of a number of warning shots, using words and phrases such as 'of concern' and 'serious', and also how the doctor uses cues from the patient to pace the giving of information. Subsequently, the doctor allows the patient time to start absorbing the information and encourages them to express their feelings and concerns. When the patient is ready, the discussion moves on to addressing these concerns and discussing the next step, the management plan. Again, the patient is encouraged to ask questions, their understanding of the situation is checked and the outcome of the consultation summarised. An offer would then be made for a further opportunity to continue the discussion and a point of contact established for concerns arising in the meantime. Some services offer an audiotape or written summary of the conversation. A summary of the discussion must be recorded in the patient notes and communicated to other key healthcare professionals involved in immediate patient care, such as the general practitioner. This approach highlights how communication is a *process* rather than a one-off event.

The importance of communication with family members or close friends of the patient is fundamental to palliative care. Such discussions must be with the permission of competent patients. Sometimes, family members insist on information being withheld from the patient for various reasons, but usually in an attempt to protect the patient from distress. Experience has shown that this is nearly always the 'wrong' thing to do. While acknowledging the insights of family members, healthcare professionals can tactfully help family to see that such collusion can add to the patient's distress. They usually pick up on non-verbal cues and can lose trust in their carers, are prevented from making informed choices, will often be aware of the progress of their physical condition and will expect answers sooner or later.

How to learn communication skills

> *Communication skills are not an optional add-on extra; without appropriate communication skills, our knowledge and intellectual efforts are easily wasted.*
> Silverman *et al.*[52]

The 'innate' skills of healthcare professionals do not seem to be sufficient to identify patient concerns, picking up on only about 40% of the issues of importance to patients,[72,73] largely physical symptoms. Communication skills training can help professionals to identify concerns, and help patients and carers to find strategies to resolve problems or to adapt to them, with the aim of reducing emotional and physical distress.

Different approaches to teaching communications skills in cancer care have evolved over the past two decades. The format of a 2- to 3-day small group, workshop-based course, sometimes residential and often multiprofessional, is common. Such courses, which use interaction and reflection as well as practise and refining of skills with immediate feedback in a supportive environment, became a popular option for those specialising in cancer and palliative care in the 1990s. The Maguire approach to acquiring communication skills[60] encourages participants to recognise barriers to disclosure of concerns and to overcome them. Participants are shown how to pick up and respond to cues, and to encourage patients to talk about their perceptions and emotional responses to events. The use of tentative, educated guesses to uncover undisclosed concerns, and the use of summarising and checking patient understanding, is also taught. Skills learned are applied to differing scenarios such as anger, denial, collusion and patients who are withdrawn.

Some evaluations of the efficacy of such courses have produced inconclusive results,[74] partly as a result of the difficulty in identifying suitable outcome measures in such a complex field with many interacting variables. However, some are more encouraging regarding the benefits of such training,[75,76] where patient disclosures increase following training and this improvement is maintained at six months.[76] Practically, the main drawback to such courses is they are both time and labour intensive, with too few qualified trainers to meet current demand for training. Other methods of teaching communication skills, such as shorter inter-active courses with larger groups, supervision in clinical practice, informal apprenticeship and shadowing, and lecture-based formats, are widespread. How-ever, formal evaluation of efficacy is often lacking for the reasons already stated. It is also thought that training that does not include some form of 'safe skills practice', i.e. role play, observation or feedback, merely raises awareness but does not cause a change in practice. It is hoped that changes to medical undergraduate curricula with regard to communications skills training will make a positive difference to clinicians' practice in the future.

What strategies have been tried regarding communication in heart failure?

Good communication encompasses the availability of clear, 'readable' informa-tion at the right time and in the right place, the application of such information through education, and the knowledge, skills and attitudes to facilitate decision making for the individual patient. Information and education are largely beyond the scope of this chapter. However, it should be noted that formal education and support interventions extending beyond the hospital setting can reduce adverse clinical outcomes and costs for patients with heart failure.[77] Comprehensive re-views of education and heart failure are available (e.g. Stromberg[78]).

The emerging literature in communication and heart failure is based largely on research of patient perceptions and concerns, and is more suggestive of strategies to be tried, rather than being descriptive or evaluative of current practice. It is a dynamic field of enquiry and some of the themes relating to language, support-ing structures, coping strategies and communication of risk will be explored here.

Language is fundamental to good communication, which is about finding out which words help and which ones hinder. Some professionals seem to have an 'innate' ability to do this well, while most learn from experience and feedback. Although colleagues may be able to help with feedback, asking patients which words they use and find helpful or otherwise is essential. Some writers have set out to 'hear' the experience of heart failure in the voices of patients and carers. The themes emerging relate to conceptions of disease, interpretation of symp-toms and effect on everyday life.

We have already mentioned that patients may not recognise the term 'heart failure' or use it in relation to themselves and that some doctors may also avoid the term because of its negative connotations.[5] That 'heart' is an emotive word for people and that the use of the word 'failure' usually connotes negative expe-riences within our culture has already been mentioned. Patients do use very negative terms in explaining their conceptions of their illness, 'such as "dead", "rubbish", "diseased", "gone completely", or "scarred tissue" to describe the condition of their heart'.[79] Whether such terms have originated from doctors, or have been thought of by patients, is unclear. There is also the situation where patients pick up terms from other patients while waiting to see the professional, or after a consultation. Such 'second-hand' knowledge may not relate to their disease state and could be misleading to them.

Choice of language can create a dilemma for professionals. The use of medical terms may ensure openness within the consultation, but when used, can result in negative emotions.[48] To avoid such reactions Tayler and Ogden go on to explain that professionals may resort to the use of euphemisms, which they may feel to be 'more neutral and less emotive'.[48] Their research, carried out among patients with heart failure in primary care, found that this appeared to be borne out in clinical practice. Use of the term 'heart failure' resulted in increased levels of anxiety and depression among patients and they viewed their illness as being more serious. It may be that the professional tailors the language they use to specific situations. However, the use of euphemisms carries its own difficulties, and it may be one of the reasons why patients with heart failure have less opportunity for end-of-life planning and less understanding of their condition compared with those dying of lung cancer, for example. Indeed, the use of euphemisms has been discouraged in the field of oncology because of this problem.

Heart failure is a devastating experience and the realities of patients need to be respected. However, at times, a lack of professional sensitivity can also hinder communication, as this quotation from a general practitioner to a patient illustrates: 'You're paddling downstream to Niagara'.[30] This comment is telling, because patients may themselves use metaphors, often relating to wind and water, in describing their experience of heart failure.[80] In her qualitative study, Zambroski outlines how patients described different phases of their illness in terms of 'experiencing turbulence, navigating, and finding safe harbour' and symptoms related to 'too much water' and 'not enough wind'.[80] Understanding of heart failure in terms of impact on everyday life is evident in many qualitative studies, for example:

> '...it's hard to put into words in't, but what I understand about it is it puts me out of breath and I can't walk and can't do owt'. Male (age 70), in Horne[79]

Another group examined patient descriptors of breathlessness in heart failure, finding three dominant experiences of breathlessness, 'every day', 'worsening' and 'uncontrollable', descriptions quite distinct from medical terminology.[81] Research with patients to identify a common language with their professional carers is at an early stage, but it promises to offer a constructive basis for dialogue.

A co-ordinated service framework is necessary to facilitate good communication.[61] Such a service framework needs to describe how different professionals communicate with patients and each other, and also who will take responsibility for the communication of specific aspects of care, including an assessment of psychosocial concerns. This is likely to differ from place to place, depending on local resources and personnel. However, in most localities, it should be possible to identify a 'key worker' to take the lead in co-ordinating care across care settings (especially hospital to home). Increasingly, this co-ordinating role is taken by heart failure clinical nurse specialists. However, general practitioners, district nurses, cardiologists, medicine for the elderly physicians and specialist palliative care team members may be appropriate practitioners for certain individuals in certain places. As many patients experience difficulty in getting to hospital appointments, mechanisms for home assessments or telephone consultations (if appropriate) should be in place.

Coping mechanisms in the self-management of heart failure have been discussed in Chapter 6. An understanding of different models of coping is particularly important to communication in the field of chronic illnesses such as heart failure, associated with progressive symptoms which seriously limit everyday life and patient choices. When giving patients news that will impact negatively on their hopes and quality of life, it is vital to be able to understand and to convey some means by which patients and their carers may be able to absorb this information and 'recentre' themselves in the light of the new information.

Everyday clinical conversations happening in the routine process of care can be a vehicle for complex discussions, including forgoing life support.[21] Such conversations, progressing through patient perception of the situation to thoughts about diagnosis, prognosis and possible treatments, may be demanding and difficult for sick patients, but appear to be well tolerated, even valued, particularly by most (but not all) patients if a family member is present:[21]

> *Within 10–20 minutes of conversation most patients seemed to be ready to talk about fundamental questions of life and death. It was also quite easy to get an idea of both the patient's values and his or her understanding of medical issues. For example, their knowledge about CPR was often very poor… no one said that they had been troubled by the conversation itself. Many patients approved. They also emphasised that it is the doctors' duty to give such information to their patients.*
> Löfmark and Nilstun[21]

Such conversations also help to clarify personal treatment goals for individual patients and wishes for future direction of care and involvement of those close to the patient in decision making.[23] Others advocate the taking of an ethics history as part of a routine clerking, including attitudes towards, and preferences for, end-of-life care, preferred model for participation in decision making, the existence of advance directives and preferences for relatives to receive information.[82]

More information and discourses from the everyday practice of clinical nurse specialists working with patients with heart failure would be informative. Each will be learning and adapting strategies from which other professionals could learn. Mike Connolly, nurse consultant in palliative care and national clinical lead of the Heart Improvement Programme, provides some of this richness in a personal account of his own practice. He highlights the fundamental principles of 'patient-centred care', not least that the patient is 'an untapped source of solutions and ways forward' and that patients can be greatly empowered by approaches that place them firmly in control of their care. He works by negotiation where, first, a patient agrees to explore their situation and second, where both patient and nurse work together to find solutions:

> *Of course I can't fix all your problems. I may actually not be able to help at all but I'd like to try if you want me to. It may be that if we put our two heads together we can make some sense of your situation and get you back to coping and feeling something like yourself again.*
> Connolly (personal account to editors, 2005)

Such an approach requires time (40 minutes plus). Connolly advocates starting with an exploration of what the patient perceives their strengths to be and how they have coped with previous difficulties, before progressing to current problems and any thoughts the patient might have about addressing these problems. He advises against starting with a formal medical history, as this might set a medical agenda and be a less effective use of time if the aim of the session is to explore psychosocial concerns and coping mechanisms. Connolly describes the single most useful question he has learned as 'Who were you before you were ill?', admitting that it takes many patients by surprise but can be a valuable tool for uncovering hopes, strengths, coping styles and self-esteem. Subsequent listing of current problems often helps patients to recognise why they can feel so overwhelmed and can be a springboard for moving forward to identify realistic goals and actions.

Communication of risk and uncertainty is a current focus of communication research. Getting communication of risk and uncertainty right is crucial to partnership models of healthcare. Currently, it is beset with difficulties. Patients need to be as informed as possible for partnerships to be real. However, little is known about how to present risk and to communicate and live with uncertainty as positively as possible. Risk information can be presented in many ways, including absolute risk, relative risk, percentages, odds and fractions, often all in the same consultation.[31] This is confounded by the fact that the data are usually derived from clinical trials with strict inclusion criteria, often excluding the very group of patients to which the individual patient belongs. Early work suggests that different mathematical representations are understood to a lesser or greater extent than others, but that there is wide variance between individuals. There is also the question of 'Risk of what?'. Doctors are likely to be focusing on risk of mortality and morbidity, whereas the patient's focus perspective may be on the likelihood of treatment restoring quality of life.[83] This represents very much a work in progress, but research in this area may yield practically useful results.

Advance directives (living wills) are formal advance statements made by a person to convey their values and preferences in relation to future medical care in the event that the person loses the capacity to decide or communicate how they wish to be treated. A competent adult's advance refusal of a specific treatment (e.g. cardiopulmonary resuscitation) has legal force (case law and Mental Capacity Act 2005[84]). Advance directives may be written or verbal. Much is written about advance directives, but with the exception of DNR orders, they are rarely used, for a number of reasons. First, few people complete them.[17] Second, to be valid, the doctor needs to be sure that these were the wishes of this particular patient, that they were competent to make this particular decision at the time of writing the directive, that the directive refers specifically to the decision in question and that there is no evidence of the patient having changed their mind in the interim or having been subject to coercion. Such evidence may not be available, particularly if a patient is admitted as an emergency, and specific situations can rarely be predicted in sufficient detail to cover the reality at hand. However, the concept of considering preferences for future care and conveying these to carers and professionals, as well as family and friends, is an important principle in palliative care. Discussion and recording of wishes both for and against likely treatment modalities, in the context of individual beliefs and values, is a key part of palliative care assessment. It is a valuable tool for enhancing communication within a group of patients for whom competence for decision making may decline with increasing frailty and disease progression. Such conversations usually take place during everyday clinical care. Knowledge of patients' values and beliefs also guide best-interest decisions when unforeseen events occur.

Future strategies in heart failure practice: general advice and specific situations

General advice

The difficulties encountered in caring for patients with heart failure and their families have been explored. Good communications skills benefit patients, carers and professionals, and need not impact negatively on time management. In practical terms, how can those involved in the management of heart failure patients adapt and improve their practice to address the concerns which have been discussed?

> 'I was told all the way through what was going to happen and why. And I think it's very important for people that one knows exactly what is going on.'
> Female cardiac patient, Kennelly and Bowling[83]

Warmth and empathy in communication are always appreciated. However, patient expectations of the relationship differ, and this needs to be identified and negotiated.

> Communication is not just about breaking bad news… it is much more. Communication is about relationship – the relationships we establish and build with our patients that make the other elements of eliciting and imparting information possible.
> Tiernan[85]

There are a number of strategies which are best avoided.[56] The 'velvet-covered hand-grenade' approach, where jargon is used to avoid open discussion of the real problem and to disguise bad news, can cause confusion and resentment. The 'hit and run' tactic, where information is given to a patient without opportunity for discussion, leaves no room for negotiation. Finally, the 'give it straight' approach in response to a question can also be harmful, as it is better to explore why the patient has asked the question and to discover what they want to know before responding.

Finally, it can be difficult to judge when it is best to initiate conversations about specific concerns, such as end-of-life care or stopping treatment. Transition points have been mentioned, and in heart failure these are often when the patient's disease progresses from one 'stage', e.g. NYHA class II, to the next. Another useful tactic is for the professional to consider the question 'Would I be surprised if this patient died within the next six to 12 months?'. If the answer is 'no', it may or may not be appropriate to approach certain topics. Comprehensive assessment, covering physical, psychosocial, quality of life and spiritual domains, would be appropriate at key transition points in the patient's illness. This could be carried out by any of the professionals involved with a patient, but decisions regarding the direction of future care are usually agreed between the patient and their doctor. Concerns, wishes and goals identified in such an assessment can lead to discussion about end-of-life care in general, and incorporate specific management decisions such as resuscitation status, advance directives and withdrawal of medical treatment. At these points, the introduction of the concept of palliative care can be appropriate. The important point to remember, again, is that communication is a *process*, not a single event.

Box 7.1 Key points to consider when communicating important issues (adapted from Kaye[56])

- Encourage the patient to bring their carer if wished
- Ensure sufficient time and privacy if at all possible
- Make sure you know the facts
- Give patient warning that the discussion is important
- Establish what the patient already knows
- Be open and honest
- Explain further if the patient wishes
- Listen to concerns and allow expression of emotion
- Involve patient and carer in decision making
- Maintain hope wherever possible
- Avoid premature or unrealistic reassurance
- It is always possible to offer the patient something: symptom control, psychological support or practical help
- Summarise the discussion
- Provide a point of contact, e.g. nurse specialist

Specific situations

Breaking bad news

Breaking bad news can be one of the most challenging tasks faced by healthcare professionals.

> *Bad news can be defined as any information that drastically alters a patient's view of their future for the worse.*
> Kaye[56]

If done well, breaking bad news can strengthen the relationship between patient and professional and contribute positively to the partnership of managing their disease. Sometimes patients cannot understand what they have been told, use denial as a protective mechanism or become angry with the professional.[86] Such anger may also be directed at themselves, at God, or cause them to question the 'fairness' of life.

To communicate bad news is important to maintain trust and reduce uncertainty for the patient, to prevent hope regarding their disease which is inappropriate, to allow them time to adjust to their changing condition and to prevent a conspiracy of silence regarding their health.[56]

Prognosis

Prognostication is difficult and understudied,[7] as well as being unpredictable (*see* Chapter 4). Patients' beliefs that they are approaching the end of their life is strongly associated with the desire to discuss prognosis,[27] and avoiding such discussions serves only to increase the patient's distress.[87] Delay in raising the subject of prognosis can delay the diagnosis of dying, and the patient is denied the opportunity to recognise that the end of their life is approaching.[32]

As a result of a failure to prognosticate, let alone prognosticate accurately, patients may die deaths they deplore in locations they despise. They may seek noxious chemotherapy rather than good palliative care, enrol in clinical or experimental therapy that offer more benefit to the researchers than to themselves, or reassure loved ones that it is not yet time to pay a visit – only to lapse into a coma before there is time to say good-bye.
Christakis[88]

Many patients are unable or unwilling to consider the future when they are well and relatively symptom-free. The subject is often raised during periods of decompensation, when patients are acutely unwell. The relevance of prognosis may diminish when patients respond to medical interventions and their conditions improve.

'We know that half of people with heart failure like yours will die in the next year. We will work together to try to help you become one of the people that lives longer than that.'
Pantilat and Steimle[23]

Prognosis is best presented to patients as a 'range estimate... with caveats'[23] given the degree of uncertainty involved. Professionals should present the situation clearly and simply, outlining the stage in their illness the patient has reached, with some communication of risk, using simple statistics if possible. Options for treatment, care and palliation of symptoms should be included in such discussions. As prognosis becomes shorter, it may be useful to use such terms as 'weeks to months', 'days to weeks' or 'hours to days'[23] to clearly convey the patient's situation to them and to their family.

Implantable cardioverter defibrillators

ICDs are used in heart failure in an attempt to prevent premature death due to arrhythmia. Their use may also prolong the dying process and make it more distressing.[89] Once such a device is inserted, discussion regarding its deactivation can be difficult as the patient's condition progresses and the end of life approaches. Goldstein *et al.*[89] reported that only 27% of carers reported that professionals had discussed deactivating ICDs.

Guidelines for discussion of ICDs with patients and their families have been produced.[90] The implications of both inserting and deactivating the device should be discussed prior to its insertion, together with consideration of advantages and disadvantages. Specifically, the situation where the patient's overall condition has deteriorated should be discussed, including the burden the ICD may then represent.

Cardiopulmonary resuscitation

The opinions and wishes of patients regarding resuscitation are not always sought[32] and the decision not to attempt resuscitation is taken on their behalf by professionals. This decision is not always communicated to the patient or their family.[91]

Guidance has been issued from many medical representative and regulatory organisations to assist professionals in making decisions regarding CPR.[92,93] As with prognosis, timing of such a discussion can be variable, but inclusion of patients and carers can act as a catalyst for discussion of future care. It has been shown, however, that patients' views on whether to agree to CPR are influenced by realistic assessments about the probability of their survival.[94]

Discussions about CPR often take place between professionals and the patient's family, as the patient may be too unwell to participate. For family members to act as surrogate decision makers and reach an informed decision, they have to be provided with all the relevant information. Approaching the subject with concern and sensitivity can reduce distress for professional, patient and carer. Communication of the patient's condition, their estimated prognosis and the predicted success of resuscitation, together with its associated negative aspects, are all important. Even when well informed, relatives can feel that they are imposing a 'death sentence' on their relative by agreeing to DNAR, and reassurance must be given that this is not the case.

Advance directives

Advance directives, as we have seen, are not the panacea for all concerns regarding future care. They are a useful tool, but ultimately do not replace discussion with patients and their carers to develop an overall picture of their wishes and preferences. Advance directives can be oral or written and discussions should focus on the patient's values and goals.[23] The professional must emphasise to the patient that considering an advance directive does not mean that treatment is being stopped. It is merely an indication of the patient's preferences for their *future* treatment and care.

> 'If you were to get so sick that you could not talk to me directly, whom should I talk with to help me make decisions about your medical care?'
> Pantilat and Steimle[23]

Palliative care

Palliative care has been mentioned throughout this chapter. Often, when patients are referred to palliative care services, discussions regarding the future direction of care have already taken place. This process of communication can continue with the involvement of palliative care specialists, whose role is to support and facilitate the patient's care and to share care with heart failure specialists and/or general practitioners.

Death and dying

The reality of *living* with advanced heart failure can mean that thoughts of approaching death may not be considered by the patient.[7] However, as Ellershaw and Ward state, 'diagnosing dying is a complex process'.[95] Patients can believe that professionals are reluctant to talk about death and dying, but structured and co-ordinated end-of-life care should be available to all patients, not just those with cancer, and vehicles such as the Liverpool Care Pathway for the dying patient[96] can be a valuable resource. Care of the dying is discussed in more detail in Chapter 8.

> '…it's this sort of roller coaster type of thing and it's very difficult to give a prognosis other than "well it's his heart, it is serious you know".'
> General practitioner, in Hanratty *et al.*[61]

'But even when you're at the very end and it's the last few weeks, you still don't know whether they're going to just die suddenly now or whether over the next few weeks they're just going to gradually drift away. So that does make it difficult in trying to prepare them and their relatives for what's actually going to happen.'
Cardiologist, in Hanratty *et al.*[61]

Conclusions

Good communication in palliative care and end-of-life decision making takes time, effort and humility. It is not an easy enterprise and the learning curve can last a lifetime. However, the rewards for effort spent are great, for patients, professionals and carers. Done well, communication at this stage of life can have a profound effect on the quality of remaining life and the death of the patient, and for the bereavement experience and memories of those dear to them. Strides have been made in professional–patient communication in general practice and oncology. Learning from patients with heart failure similarly promises to be the way forward for cardiology. If 'balancing and monitoring' are the key aspects of physical care, then 'pacing and tailoring at transition points' have the potential to advance communication in heart failure.

References

1   Dias L, Chabner BA, Lynch TJ, Penson RT. Breaking bad news: a patient's perspective. *The Oncologist* 2003; **8**: 587–96.
2   Goldacre MJ, Mant D, Duncan M, Griffith M. Mortality from heart failure in an English population, 1979–2003: study of death certification. *J Epidem Comm Health* 2005; **59**: 782–4.
3   Schaufelberger M, Swedberg K, Köster M, Rosén M, Rosengren A. Decreasing one-year mortality and hospitalization rates for heart failure in Sweden: data from the Swedish Hospital Discharge Registry 1988 to 2000. *Eur Heart Journal* 2004; **25**: 300–7.
4   Addington-Hall JM, McCarthy M. Regional study of care of the dying: methods and sample characteristics. *Pall Med* 1995; **9**: 27–35.
5   Murray SA, Boyd K, Kendall M, Worth A, Benton TF. Dying of lung cancer or cardiac failure; prospective qualitative interview study of patients and their carers in the community. *BMJ* 2002; **325**: 929–33.
6   McCarthy M, Lay M, Addington-Hall JM. Dying from heart disease. *J Royal Coll Phys London* 1996; **30**: 325–8.
7   Willems DL, Hak A, Visser F, Van der Wal G. Thoughts of patients with advanced heart failure on dying. *Pall Med* 2004; **18**: 564–72.
8   Rogers AE, Addington-Hall JM, Abery AJ, McCoy ASM, Bulpitt C, Coats AJS, Gibbs JSR. Knowledge and communication difficulties for patients with chronic heart failure: qualitative study. *BMJ* 2000; **321**: 605–7.
9   Coronary Heart Disease Collaborative. *Supportive and Palliative Care for Advanced Heart Failure.* NHS Modernisation Agency, Department of Health, London, 2004.
10 Meredith C, Symonds P, Webster L, Lamont D, Pyper E, Gillis CR, Fallowfield L. Information needs of cancer patients in west Scotland: cross sectional survey of patients views. *BMJ* 1996; **313**: 724–6.
11 Fallowfield L, Jenkins V, Farewell V, Saul J, Duffy A, Eves R. Efficacy of a Cancer Research UK communication skills training model for oncologists: a randomised controlled trial. *Lancet* 2002; **359**: 650–6.

12 Hope CJ, Wu, J, Tu W, Young J, Murray MD. Association of medication adherence, knowledge and skills with emergency department visits by adults 50 years or older with congestive heart failure. *Am J Health-System Pharm* 2004; **61**: 2043–9.

13 Moser DK, Dracup K. Psychosocial recovery from a cardiac event: the influence of perceived control. *Heart and Lung* 1995; **24**: 273–80.

14 Edmonds P, Rogers A. 'If only someone had told me' – a review of the care of patients dying in hospital. *Clin Med* 2003; **3**: 149–52.

15 Beng KS. The last hours and days of life: a biopsychosocial-spiritual model of care. *Asia Pacific Fam Med* 2004; **4**: 1–3.

16 Hopper SV, Fischback RL. Patient–physician communication when blindness threatens. *Patient Ed Couns* 1989; **14**: 69–79.

17 Formiga F, Chivite D, Ortega C, Casas S, Ramon JM, *et al.* End-of-life preferences in elderly patients admitted for heart failure. *QJM: An Int J Med* 2004; **97**: 803–8.

18 McCarthy M, Addington-Hall J. Communication and choice in dying from heart disease. *J Royal Soc Med* 1997; **90**: 128–31.

19 Wotton K, Borbasi S, Redden M. When all else has failed: nurses' perception of factors influencing palliative care for patients with end-stage heart failure. *J Cardiovasc Nurs* 2005; **20**: 18–25.

20 Boyd KJ, Murray SA, Kendall M, Worth A, Benton TF, Clausen H. Living with advanced heart failure: a prospective, community based study of patients and their carers. *Eur J Heart Fail* 2004; **6**: 585–91.

21 Löfmark R, Nilstun T. Not if, but how: one way to talk to patients about forgoing life support. *Postgrad Med J* 2000; **76**: 26–8.

22 Gibbs LME, Addington-Hall JM, Gibbs JSR. Dying from heart failure: lessons from palliative care. *BMJ* 1998; **317**: 961–2.

23 Pantilat SZ, Steimle AE. Palliative care for patients with heart failure. *JAMA* 2004; **291**: 2476–82.

24 Stewart K. Discussing cardiopulmonary resuscitation with patients and relatives. *Postgrad Med J* 1995; **71**: 585–9.

25 Mackillop WJ, Stewart WE, Ginsburg AD, Stewart SS. Cancer patients' perceptions of their disease and its treatment. *BJC* 1988; **58**: 355–8.

26 Weeks JC, Cook EF, O'Day SJ, Peterson LM, Wenger N, Reding D, Harrell FE, Kussin P, Dawson NV, Connors Jr AF, Lynn J, Phillips RS. Relationship between cancer patients' predictions of prognosis and their treatment preferences. *JAMA* 1998; **279**: 1709–14.

27 Fried TR, Bradley EH, O'Leary J. Prognosis communication in serious illness: perceptions of older patients, caregivers, and clinicians. *J Am Ger Soc* 2003; **51**: 1398–403.

28 Kutner JS, Steiner JF, Corbett KK, Jahnigen DW, Barton PL. Information needs in terminal illness. *Soc Sci Med* 1999; **48**: 1341–52.

29 Leydon GM, Boulton M, Moynihan C, Jones A, Mossman J, Boudioni M, McPherson K. Cancer patients' information needs and information seeking behaviour: in depth interview study. *BMJ* 2000; **320**: 909–13.

30 Murray SA, Boyd K, Sheikh A. Palliative care in chronic illness. *BMJ* 2005; **330**: 611–12.

31 Dudley N. Importance of risk communication and decision making in cardiovascular conditions in older patients: a discussion paper. *Qual Health Care* 2001; **10**(Suppl I): i19–i22.

32 Gibbs JSR. Heart disease. In: Addington-Hall JM, Higginson IJ (eds). *Palliative Care for Non-cancer Patients.* Oxford University Press, Oxford, 2005, pp 31–2.

33 Wenger NK. Quality of life: can it and should it be assessed in patients with heart failure? *Cardiol* 1989; **76**: 391–8.

34 Freedland KE, Carney RM, Rich MW, Caracciolo A, Krotenberg JA, Smith LJ, Sperry J. Depression in elderly patients with congestive heart failure. *J Ger Psych* 1991; **24**: 59–71.

35 Koenig HG. Depression in hospitalised older patients with congestive heart failure. *Gen Hosp Psych* 1998; **20**: 29–43.

36 Frasure-Smith N, Lesperance F, Talajic M. Depression following myocardial infarction. *JAMA* 1993; **270**: 1819–25.

37 Rabins PV, Harvis K, Koven S. High fatality rates of late life depression associated with cardiovascular disease. *J Aff Dis* 1985; **9**: 165–7.

38 Carney RM, Rich MW, Freedland KE, Saini J, teVelde A, Simeone C, Clark K. Major depressive disorder predicts cardiac events in patients with coronary artery disease. *Psychosom Med* 1988; **50**: 627–33.

39 Carney RM, Freedland KE, Eisen SA, Rich MW, Jaffe AS. Major depression and medication adherence in elderly patients with coronary artery disease. *Health Psych* 1995; **14**: 88–90.

40 Dunbar J. Predictors of patient adherence: patient characteristics. In: Shumaker SA, Schron EB, Ockene JK (eds). *The Handbook of Health Behaviour Change*. Springer, New York, 1998, pp 348–60.

41 Hawthorne MH, Hixon ME. Functional status, mood disturbance and quality of life in patients with heart failure. *Prog Cardiovasc Nursing* 1994; **9**: 22–32.

42 Maricle RA, Hosenpud JD, Norman DJ, Woodbury A, Pantley GA, Cobanoglu AM, Starr A. Depression in patients being evaluated for heart transplantation. *Gen Hosp Psych* 1989; **11**: 418–24.

43 Wehby D, Brenner PS. Perceived learning needs of patients with heart failure. *Heart Lung* 1997; **28**: 31–40.

44 Franciosa JA, Wilen M, Ziesche S, Cohn JN. Survival in men with severe chronic left ventricular failure due to either coronary artery disease or idiopathic dilated cardiomyopathy. *Am J Cardiol* 1983; **51**: 831–6.

45 Gradman A, Deedwania P, Cody R, Massie B, Packer M, Pitt B, Goldstein S. Predictors of total mortality and sudden death in mild to moderate heart failure. Captopril – digoxin study group. *J Am Coll Cardiol* 1989; **14**: 564–70.

46 Kjekshus J. Arrhythmias and mortality in congestive heart failure. *Am J Cardiol* 1990; **65**: 421–81.

47 CONSENSUS Trial Study Group. Effects of enalapril on mortality in severe congestive heart failure. Results of the Cooperative North Scandinavian Enealapril Survival Study (CONSENSUS). *New Eng J Med* 1997; **316**: 1429–35.

48 Tayler M, Ogden J. Doctors' use of euphemisms and their impact of patients' beliefs about health: an experimental study of heart failure. *Pat Ed Counseling* 2005; **57**: 321–6.

49 Christakis NA, Iwashyna TJ. Attitude and self-reported practice regarding prognostication in a national sample of internists. *Arch Int Med* 1998; **158**: 2389–95.

50 Lamont EB, Christakis NA. Complexities in prognostication in advanced cancer. *JAMA* 2003; **290**: 98–104.

51 Kurtz S, Silverman J, Draper J. *Teaching and Learning Communication Skills in Medicine* (2e). Radcliffe Publishing Ltd, Oxford, 2005.

52 Silverman J, Kurtz S, Draper J. *Skills for Communicating with Patients* (2e). Radcliffe Publishing Ltd, Oxford, 2005, p 7.

53 Makoul G. Communication skills education in medical school and beyond. *msJAMA* 2003; **289**: 93.

54 Emanuel EJ, Emanuel LL. Four models of the physician-patient relationship. *JAMA* 1992; **267**: 2221–6.

55 Randall F, Downie RS. *Palliative Care Ethics: a companion for all specialties* (2e). Oxford University Press, Oxford, 1999.

56 Kaye P. *Breaking Bad News: a ten step approach*. EPL, Northampton, 1996, p 3.

57 Statham H, Dimavicius J. Commentary: How do you give the bad news to parents? *Birth* 1992; **19**: 103–4.

58 Buckman R. Breaking bad news: why is it still so difficult? *BMJ* 1984; **288**: 1597–9.

59 Speck P. Communication skills. Breaking bad news. *Nursing Times* 1991; **87**: 24–6.

60 Maguire P, Pitceathley C. Key communication skills and how to acquire them. *BMJ* 2002; **325**: 697–700.

61 Hanratty B, Hibbert D, Mair F, May C, Ward C, Capewell S, Litva A, Corcoran G. Doctors' perceptions of palliative care for heart failure: focus group study. *BMJ* 2002; **325**: 581–5.

62 Oken D. What to tell cancer patients: a study of medical attitudes. *JAMA* 1961; **175**: 1120–8.

63 Charlton RC. Breaking bad news. *Med J Aus* 1992; **157**: 615–21.

64 Goldberg RJ. Disclosure of information to adult cancer patients: issues and update. *J Clin Oncol* 1984; **2**: 948–55.

65 Woodward LJ, Pamies RL. The disclosure of the diagnosis of cancer. *Primary Care* 1992; **19**: 657–63.

66 National Institute for Clinical Excellence (2004). *Guidelines on Cancer Services: improving supportive and palliative care for adults with cancer.* NICE, London, 2004.

67 Fallowfield LJ, Jenkins VA, Beveridge HA. Truth may hurt but deceit hurts more: communication in palliative care. *Pall Med* 2002; **16**: 297–303.

68 Fallowfield L, Saul J, Gilligan B. Teaching senior nurses how to teach communication skills in oncology. *Cancer Nursing* 2001; **24**: 185–91.

69 Razavi D, Delvaux N, Marchal S, Bredart A, Farvacques C, Paesmans M. The effects of a 24 hour psychological training programme on attitudes, communication skills and occupational stress in oncology: a randomised study. *Eur J Cancer* 1993; **29**: 1858–63.

70 Wilkinson S, Bailey K, Aldridge J, Roberts A. A longitudinal evaluation of a communication skills programme. *Pall Med* 1999; **13**: 341–8.

71 Buckman R. *How to Break Bad News: a guide for health care professionals.* Papermac, London, 1994.

72 Parle M, Jones B, Maguire P. Maladaptive coping and affective disorders in cancer patients. *Psychol Med* 1996; **26**: 735-44.

73 Heaven CM, Maguire P. Disclosure of concerns by hospice patients and their identification by nurses. *Pall Med* 1997; **11**: 283–90.

74 Fellowes D, Wilkinson S, Moore P. Communication skills training for health care professionals working with cancer patients, their families and/or carers (Cochrane Review). *The Cochrane Database of Systematic Reviews* 2004, Issue 2. Art. No.: CD003751. DOI: 10.1002/14651858/CD003751.pub2., 2004.

75 Aspegren K. Teaching and learning communication skills in medicine – a review with quality grading of articles. *Medical Teacher* 1999; **21**: 563–70.

76 Maguire P, Booth K, Elliott C, Jones B. Helping health professionals involved in cancer care acquire key interviewing skills – the impact of workshops. *Eur J Cancer* 1996; **32**: 1486–9.

77 Krumholz HM, Amatruda J, Smith GL, Mattera JA *et al.* Randomized trial of an education and support intervention to prevent readmission of patients with heart failure. *J Am Coll Cardiol* 2002; **39**: 83–9.

78 Stromberg A. Educating nurses and patients to manage heart failure. *Eur J Cardiovasc Nursing* 2002; **1**: 33–40.

79 Horne G. Removing the boundaries: palliative care for patients with heart failure. *Pall Med* 2004; **18**: 291–6.

80 Zambroski CH. Qualitative analysis of living with heart failure. *Heart Lung* 2003; **32**: 32–40.

81 Edmonds PM, Rogers A, Addington-Hall JM, McCoy A *et al.* Patient descriptors of breathlessness in heart failure. *Int J Cardiol* 2005; **98**: 61–6.

82 Sayers GM, Barratt D, Gothard C, Onnie C, Perera S *et al.* The value of taking an 'ethics history'. *J Med Eth* 2001; **27**: 114–17.

83 Kennelly C, Bowling A. Suffering in deference: a focus group study of older cardiac patients' preferences for treatment and perceptions of risk. *Qual Health Care* 2001; **10**(Suppl I): i23–8.

84 HM Government. *Mental Capacity Act 2005.* The Stationery Office, London, 2005.

84 Tiernan E. Communication training for professionals. *Supp Care Cancer* 2003; **11**: 758–62.

86 Lloyd-Williams M. Breaking bad news to patients and relatives. *BMJ* 2002; **325**: s11–12.

87 Stedford A. *Facing Death.* Heinemann, London, 1984.

88 Christakis NA. *Death Foretold: prophecy and prognosis in medical care.* University of Chicago Press, Chicago IL, 1999.

89 Goldstein NE, Lampert R, Bradley E, Lynn J, Krumholz HM. Management of implantable cardioverter defibrillators in end-of-life care. *Ann Int Med* 2004; **141**: 835–8.

90 Harrington MD, Luebke DL, Lewis WR, Aulisio MP, Johnson NJ (2004). Fast Facts and Concepts #112. *Implantable Cardioverter Defibrillator (ICD) at End of Life.* End-of-Life Physician Education Resource Center (www.eperc.mcw.edu).

91 Löfmark R, Nilstun T. Do-not-resuscitate orders – should the patients be informed? *J Int Med* 1997; **241**: 421–5.

92 British Medical Association. *Withholding and Withdrawing Life-prolonging Medical Treatment: guidance for decision making* (2e). BMJ Books, London, 2002.

93 General Medical Council. *Withholding and Withdrawing Life-prolonging Treatments: good practice in decision-making.* General Medical Council, London, 2002.

94 Murphy DJ, Burrows D, Santilli S. The influence of the probability of survival on patients' preferences regarding cardiopulmonary resuscitation. *New Eng J Med* 1994; **330**: 545–9.

95 Ellershaw J, Ward C. Care of the dying patient: the last hours or days of life. *BMJ* 2003; **326**: 30–4.

96 Ellershaw J, Wilkinson S (eds). *Care of the Dying: a pathway to excellence.* Oxford University Press, Oxford, 2003.

Chapter 8

Care of the patient dying from heart failure

Clare Littlewood and Miriam Johnson

Care of the dying is an integral part of the healthcare professional's role. The majority of general practitioners see it as one of their most important tasks, and one from which they gain much job satisfaction.[1] Carers are often very appreciative of good care given, but also distressed when this is lacking. And yet, despite its universal inevitability, many fears and taboos still persist about death and dying, and these inhibit the discussion of end-of-life issues by healthcare professionals. These fears are based on societal norms and they result in less than ideal deaths, even for those whose death is anticipated.

A new way of dying

As society learns how to stave off more and more diseases, an increasing proportion of the population are living into their eighties and beyond. Many now believe that medical science will provide a cure for anything that ails them, including old age and death. As a consequence, dying in society has moved from expected, open and at home to 'abnormal', hidden and in hospitals. Subsequently, with the removal of death from everyday life, families have lost the knowledge of how to care for and even relate to the dying person. The dying process is also often linked with fear. Hinton,[2] as far back as 1963, noted that there were irrational fears in our culture that exaggerate the horrors of death. Palliative care has encouraged healthcare professionals to be more accepting of death, but the charge of creeping medicalisation of dying has also been levelled at palliative care.[3] This is particularly relevant for patients with advanced heart failure, where optimal medical management approximately doubles life expectancy. Recent research into biventricular pacing on top of medical therapy suggests that the previously bleak prognosis of chronic heart failure can be improved even further.[4] Under these circumstances it can be very hard for both doctor and patient to accept that dying is inevitable.

Dying at home

If asked, most patients express a preference to die at home, and yet only a quarter of cancer patients achieve this,[5] and even fewer, if overall deaths are considered.[6]

Care of the patient dying from heart failure

In order to die at home, patients and carers need a sense of security from the team delivering that care, good symptom control, adequate support and open communication about the aim of care. The changing face of primary care, a new contract and subsequent disappearance of 24-hour cover by general practitioners has led to difficulties providing secure out-of-hours care for the terminally ill. Patients with heart failure often experience chest pain in their dying process, which for many telephone nurse-led triage systems will be dealt with as a medical emergency necessitating an emergency 'blue flashing light' ambulance and attendance at the Accident and Emergency department.

Primary care remains keen to address these problems and the will to remain involved is helped by frameworks of care such as the Gold Standards (GSF) (also discussed in Chapter 10).[7,8] This was developed as a tool to aid primary care teams improve community-delivered palliative care by facilitating better team co-ordination and communication, with particular regard to anticipatory and out-of-hours care. Although initially designed for use with patients suffering from cancer, it is readily transferable to those dying from non-cancer-related diseases such as heart failure. With our ageing population, the number of family members available to give assistance to healthcare professionals with the delivery of home-based care is reduced. Home palliative care is often not possible without the support of these unpaid caregivers. Estimates of the current value of the support given by carers have been around the same level as the total UK spending on health, about £57 billion in 2001–02.[9] With fewer and fewer non-professional primary caregivers for heart failure and insufficient professional carers to plug the gap (indeed there are areas in UK that do not have access to 24-hour district nursing service), establishing 24-hour care at home without further resources is not a reality. Results from Canada show that de-institutionalisation of services from hospitals for terminally ill cancer patients to care at home and hospices resulted in a neutral cost saving because of decreased acute bed usage with increased use of more appropriate settings for their care.[10] If this is to become a reality in this country, then healthcare commissioners need to develop a seamless service to channel resources to where they are needed most to enable patients to die in their preferred place of care. The GSF is a good start, and an analysis of phase 4 has shown an increase in the numbers of patient able to do so.[8]

Dying in hospital

However, all too often, the care of the dying, especially those with prolonged illness trajectories like heart failure who have well-established links with hospital care, die in the hospital setting. Again, because of sudden decompensations, which may be triggered by reversible causes, or which may respond to optimisation of treatment and from which the patient may recover, acute hospital admission is likely unless discussions have been made to the contrary in advance and alternative supports put in place. As discussed, this can be difficult, as it can be hard to know which decompensation will be a terminal event. Studies have shown that care of the dying in hospital can be poor. Mills et al.[11] in 1994 reported their findings 13 years after their initial research, showing that basic interventions for dying patients were often not provided. Oral hygiene was poor and little assistance was given to encourage eating or drinking. A later study[12] found similar evidence of distancing tactics used by professionals. It found that 73% of relatives were dissatisfied with information given and the manner in which it was given.

In 2005, care of the dying in the hospital setting remains difficult to do well. The increasing throughput of patients results in greater pressure on bed occupancy, with almost a quarter of hospital bed-days taken up by patients in the last year of life. Busy hospital wards focus on 'cure' and discharge, and sometimes view dying patients as 'failure', with the risk that nursing and medical teams withdraw, becoming less and less involved as the patient comes closer to death. Vital signs and arterial blood gas sampling may continue, but basic nursing procedures such as mouth care are often omitted. Attention to care of the family and privacy may be missing. The care of the sickest group of patients is often left to the most junior doctor and nurse of the team.

It is for these reasons that a care pathway for the dying patient was developed by a multiprofessional team of doctors and nurses in Liverpool.[13,14] This pathway uses the best practice principles of care delivered by hospices in a format that is transferable to other settings. It is a tool that has been adopted nationally both by the *NHS Cancer Plan*,[15] NICE guidance[16] and Gold Standards Framework[7] as a way of improving the care of dying patients.

Dying in hospice

Hospice care of the dying is thought to be the gold standard. However, despite there being over 535,990 deaths in England and Wales in 2003, of which 26% were due to cancers[17] and 38% were due to circulatory disease, less than 1% of patients with heart disease were admitted to a hospice for end-of-life care. Hospices arose out of a desire to improve the care that cancer patients received under the NHS. Most were set up outside the auspices of the NHS and even now, on average, only receive approximately one-third of their income from the NHS, the rest provided by charitable fund raising. This has led to a fear by some of current services being overrun without adequate resources and, indeed, possibly denying access to the very cancer patients they were built to deal with. Coupled with the reluctance and uncertainty of primary and secondary care teams of when to refer, access to inpatient units is low.

There is also some reluctance of specialist palliative care services to change and indeed, limit referrals to cancer and motor neurone disease alone although others have an 'open door' policy and accept all diseases. This lack of uniformity among hospices may cause confusion for patients and professionals.

Heart failure as a terminal illness

Medicine itself has not helped with the propagation of fears about death. The ever-increasing emphasis on a cure rather than care is particularly evident in the management of patients with advanced heart failure. We have seen elsewhere in the book that death and dying are often not discussed openly with patients with heart failure, who often have a poor and incomplete understanding of their illness and prognosis.

Heart failure has a poor prognosis (*see* Chapter 4);[18] a recent UK population-based study reported survival at one year from diagnosis to be as low as 62% for all age groups. Cardiovascular mortality also increases with age by 26% for every 10 years since diagnosis.

There is little doubt, therefore, that patients with advanced heart failure have limited life expectancy, and yet so few receive a chance to plan their end of life or receive supportive and palliative care.

Specialist palliative care services include inpatient, day patient, outpatient and bereavement care, as well as advisory roles, both in hospital and primary care settings. This clinical activity is supported by education, audit and research. Despite a change in emphasis from end-of life care only to earlier referral for support and rehabilitation and an increasing openness to deliver services to patients without cancer,[19] there is still a common misperception by healthcare professionals that palliative care is only for the management of patients in terminal stages of malignant disease. Thus patients with end-stage heart failure often still do not have the access to services when they come to die.

'Supportive care' is a new, all-embracing definition which may cover the needs of patients with advanced heart failure more fully and yet as Murray and Kendall state,[20] 'we must not be constrained by our inability to predict the terminal phase of disease'. Much has been written about prognostication already[21] (*see* Chapter 4) and this indeed is one of the most-quoted reasons for lack of referral to specialist palliative care services.[22]

Recognition of the 'dying phase'

It can be difficult to judge when life expectation is very limited and when a change from active treatment to terminal care is or should be considered appropriate.[23] This is compounded by a valid concern that a reversible precipitant may be overlooked. It is particularly difficult for patients awaiting transplantation, where there may be a perceived need to be kept alive at all costs in a situation where there is increasing recognition of the tensions suffered by both patient and relative.[24,25] The development of further medications and devices such as implantable cardioverter defibrillators (ICDs) and left ventricle assist devices (LVADs) has made the decision of when to stop treatment in a patient with heart failure particularly difficult. ICDs were originally developed to prevent sudden deaths in patients with life-threatening ventricular arrhythmias. They are internal devices that can monitor heart rhythms and defibrillate a patient with a shock of up to 40 joules of energy when a life-threatening rhythm is detected. Their use in patients with advanced heart failure is limited but increasing. The recognition of the dying phase under these circumstances is crucial. Inappropriate triggering in the dying phase can be distressing for both patient and carers.[26–28] It is important to address this issue early and it is argued that the patient should be counselled at insertion of such a device, that the time may come when it will need to be deactivated, that is if a patient wishes for a do-not-resuscitate (DNR) order.[29,30] This can be done temporarily with a large magnet placed over the chest wall, but as this is only effective while the magnet is present, the decision to turn the ICD off should be taken with enough time to organise for the cardiology centre that fitted the device to deactivate it using the correct telemetry equipment. Ideally, local technicians could be trained to do this, and discussion regarding local solutions in the situation where the patient is too sick to go to the nearest tertiary centre is encouraged.

The diagnosis of dying is a combination of science and art. One of the barriers may be that healthcare professionals are unsure what to do for dying patients and therefore continue with the treatment they know, thus saving the difficult and awkward problem of making the 'diagnosis of dying'.

Care pathways

Use of a care pathway for the dying patient at this point is a tool that can empower healthcare professionals to deliver evidence-based best practice. Integrated care pathways were originally developed in the USA.[31] They were developed to enable hospital palliative care teams to enable generic staff to deliver quality care of the dying and prevent deskilling. They are particularly useful for nursing care where unhelpful vital sign monitoring is replaced with prompted useful activity such as mouth and bowel care, attention to spiritual needs and family concerns. Optimal care does not necessarily have to be delivered via a pathway. It is merely one way of getting around the problems of inadequate documentation, maintaining continuity of care and promoting good team communication despite shift working, locums and the use of unfamiliar 'out-of-hours' doctors.

By using the Liverpool Care Pathway (LCP) for the dying patient many of the anticipated problems can be overcome, as it empowers teams to anticipate care and so minimise the need for unfamiliar professionals to be involved. The LCP was developed by a multiprofessional team involved in the caring process over a two-year time period. It incorporates evidence-based practice and appropriate guidelines for the commonest symptoms experienced by the dying patient.[32] For heart failure these include pain, dyspnoea, agitation, nausea and vomiting, and management of chest secretions.

The pathway then acts as a prompt for the process of care that is to be delivered with the expected outcome. Some professionals have concerns that a pathway detracts from clinical judgement. However, the LCP has inbuilt flexibility, so if one of the 'goals' is not achieved, for example it is considered in the patient's interests to continue intravenous antibiotics, then that is fine, as long as the clinical justification is documented. If the prompted goals are not achieved, the reason is documented. This deviation from expected care delivery is called a 'variance'. Thus inappropriate prescribing and poor clinical decision making is minimised.

Analysis of variance provides useful information about practice. It is important that healthcare professionals understand that variances do not necessarily mean a deficit of care, but may highlight more effective ways of delivering the care or identify educational research issues.

There are four key elements of the LCP:

1 identification of the dying patient
2 initial assessment and care

3 ongoing assessments
4 care of relatives after death.

Identification of dying patients

When a patient enters the dying phase they are usually have at least two of the following four features: bed bound, semi-conscious, can only take sips of fluid, unable to take oral medication. In addition to these observations, the multiprofessional team should be in agreement that the patient is entering the dying phase. In cancer patients, the median time to death given these criteria is two days.[33] Evidence is currently lacking in patients with heart failure, but those centres using the LCP for such patients use the same criteria without reported difficulty. There may be reluctance to place a heart failure patient on the pathway, because it is recognised that they may survive despite an acute and severe decompensation. However, if the patient subsequently stabilises (not uncommon when symptom control is achieved) and it seems that the patient will survive the episode, the patient can be taken off the pathway.

Patients with advanced heart failure who are reaching end stage usually have increasingly frequent hospitalisations characterised by worsening oedema and progressive renal failure despite optimal tolerated therapy in the absence of a reasonable cause. At this stage, discussion with the patient and carers should be encouraged and further management planned taking their wishes into account.

End-of-life decisions regarding cardiopulmonary resuscitation (CPR) and ICD devices can be finalised and the goals of care explained. The findings of the SUPPORT study suggest that these consultations around end-of-life wishes are not taking place.[34] These decisions need to have happened before starting a patient with heart failure on a dying pathway. This is of particular importance for hospices, many of which do not have resuscitation facilities. Patients may request that a pacemaker device be turned off at this stage. While this is a valid request in a competent patient for withdrawal of treatment,[28,35–37] it is not certain what the outcome would be. If the patient were pacemaker dependent, then death may be hastened by turning the rate down to the minimum 30 beats per minute. However, some may not be so, and may risk the reappearance of the very symptoms the pacemaker was put in to solve. Some argue that as death approaches, the myocardium becomes less and less responsive to pacemaker stimulation and the situation becomes irrelevant. Thus is it hard to anticipate the effect of such action on the dying process, and research on such issues would be difficult to perform.

Initial assessment and care

Once the team has decided the patient is dying then the pathway identifies that the active care should include the following.

- Review of all medication. Active measures are often continued to aid patient care, e.g. continuation of diuretics to relieve dyspnoea. Loop diuretics may be needed right up until death to help prevent severe pulmonary oedema. Venous access is often difficult at this stage and attempts to cannulate become a further cause of distress to the patient. To prevent this, or painful intramuscular injections, furosemide can be administered by continuous subcutaneous infusion via a syringe driver.[38,39] Transdermal nitrates may be useful at this stage, both to relieve any angina, and also in addition to a loop diuretic in an attempt to prevent pulmonary oedema.

- Discontinuation of non-essential medication and procedures, including inappropriate nursing interventions such as vital sign monitoring and two-hourly turns.
- Switching off ICD if not already done so.
- Anticipatory prescribing as required, medication for pain, nausea, vomiting, respiratory tract and secretions, and dyspnoea. (Symptom control measures are described in Chapter 5.)
- Ensure cultural, religious and spiritual needs of the dying patient and family are addressed.

Ongoing care of the dying heart failure patient

The Liverpool Care Pathway for the dying patient emphasises the active nature of the care of the dying, with at least four-hourly observations of the symptom control issues and the need to take appropriate action if there are any problems. There is also a prompt to assess the psychological and spiritual support given to patient and family every 12 hours.

Care of family and carers after death

Here the care focuses on the legal requirements, the support needed by families and carers immediately after death, and any special needs for care of the body.

It is usual to give a leaflet about bereavement to the family. This focuses on the feelings of the relatives that are common in bereavement and useful contact addresses for bereavement support.

Other leaflets

Research has shown that families sometimes need more information about the dying process itself. A leaflet 'Coping with the Dying'[40] has been developed by practising palliative care nurses. This, in conjunction with exploration from the multidisciplinary team, may allay some fears. Particular concerns may arise with regard to ICDs and the need to switch such devices to pacing mode in patients dying from heart failure. It is important to be clear that the reasoning behind switching off the device is seen as appropriate withdrawal of medical treatment and not euthanasia.[28] A leaflet regarding these issues may help allay these fears for both professionals and carers alike and is being developed by the LCP team.

Conclusion

A major cultural shift within both the medical profession and society in general is required if the needs of patients dying from heart failure are to be met. Care of the dying is integral to every doctor's practice, and it is imperative that these patients are not deserted. The hospice movement and specialty of palliative care has been instrumental in improving the care of the dying cancer patient. It is important that we now strive to improve the care of the patient dying from heart failure. It is no longer acceptable for doctors to say 'it's not my job' or 'there's nothing more I can do'. Potential fragmentation of care that can occur between primary and secondary care must be avoided, and a high standard of anticipatory care practised to deal with problems out of hours. Multiprofessional teamworking and the use of tools such as the LCP can help provide a consistent, well-documented high standard of care.

References

1　Lehman R. How long can I go on like this? *Br J Gen Pract* 2004; **54**: 892–3.
2　Hinton JM. The physical and mental distress of the dying. *Quart J Med* 1963; **125**:1–21.
3　Clark D. Between hope and acceptance: the medicalisation of dying. *BMJ* 2003; **324**: 905–7.
4　Clark AL. What's new in heart failure? *Medicine* 2005; **33**(10): 1–4.
5　Higginson I, Astin P, Dolan S. Where do cancer patients die? Ten year trends in the place of death of cancer patients in England. *Pall Med* 1998; **12**(5): 353–63.
6　Ellershaw J, Ward C. Care of the dying patient: the last hours or days of life. *BMJ* 2003; **326**: 30–4.
7　Thomas K. *Caring for the Dying at Home*. Radcliffe Medical Press, Oxford, 2003.
8　Samar M, Kristjanson L, Currow D *et al*. Caregiving for the terminally ill: at what cost? *Pall Med* 2005; **19**: 551–5.
9　Fassbender K, Fasinger R, Brenneis C *et al*. Utilisation and costs of the introduction of system wide palliative care in Alberta, 1993–2000. *Pall Med* 2005; **19**: 513–20.
10　Department of Health. www.goldstandardsframework.nhs.uk
11　Mills M, Davies HTO, Macrae WA. Dying in hospital. *BMJ* 1994; **309**: 583–6.
12　Rogers S, Karlsen S, Addington-Hall J. Dying for care: the experiences of terminally ill cancer patients in an inner city health district. *Pall Med* 2000; **14**(1): 53–6.
13　Ellershaw J, Wilkinson S (eds). *Care of the Dying: a pathway to excellence*. Oxford University Press, Oxford, 2004.
14　Liverpool Care Pathway for the Dying. www.lcp-mariecurie.org.uk
15　Department Of Health. *The NHS Cancer Plan*. DoH, London, 2000.
16　Improving Supportive and Palliative Care for Adults with Cancer, 2004. www.NICE.org.uk
17　Office for National Statistics. *Annual Review of the Registrar General on Deaths in England and Wales*. www.statistics.gov.uk/downloads/themehealth/HSQ28.pdf (accessed January 2006).
18　Courie M, Wood DA. Survival of patients with a new diagnosis of heart failure. *Heart* 2000; **83**: 505–10.
19　Clarke D. Originating a movement; Cicely Saunders and the development of St Christopher's Hospice 1957–67. *Morality* 1983; **4**: 43–6.
20　Murray S, Kendall M. Illness trajectories and palliative care. *BMJ* 2005; **330**: 1007–9
21　Mosterd A, Cost B, Hoes AW *et al*. The prognosis of heart failure in the general population. *Eur Heart J* 2001; **22**: 1318–27.
22　Hanratty B, Hibbert D *et al*. Doctors perceptions of palliative care for heart failure – a focus study. *BMJ* 2002; **325**: 581–5.
23　Working Party on Clinical Guidelines in Palliative Care. *Changing Gear – guidelines for managing the last days of life. The research evidence*. NCHSPCS, London, 1997.

24 Evangelista LS, Dracup K, Moser DK *et al*. Two-year follow-up of quality of life in patients referred for heart transplant. *Heart Lung* 2005; **34**: 187–93.

25 Castle H, Jones I. A long wait: how nurses can help patients through the transplantation pathway. *Prof Nurse* 2004; **19**: 37–9.

26 Nambisan V, Chao D. Dying and defibrillation: a shocking experience. *Pall Med* 2004; **18**: 482–3.

27 Goldstein NE, Lampert R, Bradley E *et al*. Management of implantable cardioverter defibrillator in end-of-life care. *Ann Intern Med* 2004: **141**: 835–8.

28 Berger JT. The ethics of deactivating implanted cardioverter defibrillators. *Ann Intern Med* 2005; **142**: 631–4.

29 Morrison LJ, Sinclair CT, Goldstein NE *et al*. Next-of kin responses and do-not-resuscitate implications for implantable cardioverter defibrillators/in response. [Letter] *Ann Intern Med* 2005; **142**: 676–7.

30 Beattie JM, Connolly MJ, Ellershaw JE. Deactivating implantable cardioverter defibrillators/in response. [Letter] *Ann Intern Med* 2005; **143**: 690.

31 Overill S. A practical guide to care pathways. *J Integr Care* 1998; **2**: 93–8.

32 Ellershaw J, Smith C, Overill S *et al*. Care of the dying; setting standards for symptom control in the last 48 hours of life. *JPSM* 2001; **21**: 12–17.

33 Adam J. The last 48 hours of life. *BMJ* 1997; **315**: 1600–3.

34 Levenson JW, McCarthy EP, Lynn J *et al*. The last six months of life for patients with congestive heart failure. *J Am Geriatric Soc* 2000; **48**: 101–9.

35 Mueller PS, Hook CC, Hayes DL. Ethical analysis of withdrawal of pacemaker or implantable cardioverter–defibrillator support at the end of life. *Mayo Clin Pract* 2003; **78**: 959–63.

36 Ross HM. Deactivating implantable cardioverter defibrillators/in response. [Letter] *Ann Intern Med* 2005; **143**: 690.

37 Berger JT. Deactivating implantable cardioverter defibrillators/in response. [Letter] *Ann Intern Med* 2005; **143**: 691

38 Verma AK, da Silva JH, Kuhl DR. Diuretic effects of subcutaneous furosemide in human volunteers: a randomised pilot study. *Ann Pharmacother* 2004; **38**: 544–9.

39 Goenaga MA. Millet M, Sanchez E *et al*. Subcutaneous furosemide. [Comment] *Ann Pharmacother* 2004; **38**: 1751.

40 Salmon I, Griffiths C, Bridson J. *Coping with Dying. Understanding the changes which occur before death.* www.lcp-mariecurie.org.uk

Chapter 9

Palliative care needs of young people with heart failure

Hayley Pryse-Hawkins

Earlier chapters have established that heart failure is a potentially malignant, chronic, debilitating condition suffered by a very large number of patients and their families. We have seen that the average age of patients with heart failure in the UK is 77, which is similar to the average age of patients with cancer. But just as with cancer, heart failure can sometimes affect children and young adults, and although the number of such individuals is much smaller, the impact of a life-threatening illness coming early in life can be devastating.

There is little written about the specific palliative needs of young people with advanced heart failure. Therefore the approach taken is descriptive rather than prescriptive. It is important to understand not only what heart failure is, but how it affects people in different stages. For the purpose of this chapter, 'young' will span the years between paediatric and geriatric provision (16–65 years). We shall also be dealing with more specifically age-related issues, such as sexuality, procreation, body image, and transition from paediatric to adult services.

The need for evidence-based care

To meet the needs of heart failure patients we will be required to provide evidence, funding and resources. Heart failure is predominantly a condition of the elderly, and associated with complex co-morbidities, which may affect patients' quality of life and prognosis equally. Traditionally, research in heart failure has used a cohort of people under 70 years and extrapolated the evidence across the heart failure population. By selecting such subjects, it is generally easier to gain consent, ethical agreement and to avoid confounding from other disease processes. With an older cohort with numerous co-morbidities it is more difficult to establish the needs and outcomes which are heart failure and not age specific. For younger patients, there are different problems: for example, the disease processes underlying their heart failure may be very rare, making recruitment difficult for particular aetiologies.

Young people with heart failure will therefore be asked to enter clinical trials and studies at all stages of their disease trajectory, but not always with a potential personal gain. This will require sensitive management and integration of palliative, cardiac and research services. Young people will need clear guidelines and supportive structures to enable them to partake in such research.

Point to consider

- There is little research specifically into the needs of younger patients with heart failure, despite younger people being most likely to be involved in research projects.

Timing of appropriate care

In contrast with many cancers, in heart failure there is not a clear pathway of care from diagnosis, through treatment, to palliation. Most cardiologists and physicians managing young people with heart failure have little palliative education or experience, and may consequently find it difficult to recognise the needs and transition phases such patients face.

Heart failure patients are more likely to die in hospital and to undergo clinical interventions in the last few weeks and days of their life.[1] This is especially so with younger patients, where hospital staff fail to recognise and accept how close to death patients are. Added to this, most health professionals will encounter only a few younger heart failure patients in their working lifetime. A third of patients admitted with decompensated heart failure die within one year of their first hospitalisation and up to 50% will be readmitted within the first six months after the initial hospitalisation. The challenge for health professionals is to identify which patients are more likely to die within the next 12 months. The 'surprise' question ('Would you be surprised if this patient died in the next 12 months?') has been adopted as a useful trigger for a palliative approach (*see* Chapter 4).

Accurately predicting outcomes, disease trajectories and death is difficult for even the most experienced doctor, even without the emotional issues of the patient being as young or younger than the professional. The emphasis in cardiology care is predominantly curative, and professionals lack the training and support required to recognise the subtle changes that may suggest a patient is dying. There is a fear of recognising and admitting there is no further intervention that can 'save' the patient. There is also a sense of helplessness and ignorance among healthcare professionals of what happens next, which make it difficult to recognise and discuss such changes.

We have seen in Chapter 4 that a large number of prognostic tools exist. Cardiac transplant assessments incorporate a variety of these tools and measures to assess suitability for transplantation. These are guides and useful reference points, but despite intensive monitoring it is usually difficult to predict which decompensation episode precedes death. However, recognising a change in functional ability, an increasing frequency of decompensations or an escalation in symptom burden may be a non-invasive trigger for considering supportive care. Staff who are trained and skilled to assess the continually changing needs of their heart failure patients will be better able to recognise when their patients are requiring supportive end-of-life rather than curative care. They will be better able to communicate this to the patient and family, and to provide appropriate information, care and resources.

Point to consider

- Despite heart failure having a poor prognosis, it can be difficult for healthcare professionals to recognise and accept that a young person cannot be cured, and is actually dying.

Healthcare professional education

A palliative care approach, with sensitive discussions and excellent channels of communication, would be helpful for most young heart failure patients, and would be best provided by involved heart failure professionals and the primary healthcare team. Many young heart failure patients require access to palliative services at some point, but only a few are likely to need continual access to specialist palliative care professionals. This relies on heart failure and primary care staff education, confidence and collaboration, as much as specialist palliative care service provision. NICE clearly endorses the importance of supportive and palliative care being a clear priority for all heart failure services.[2,3]

Patients of all ages with heart failure need clear information about heart failure, its symptoms, management and prognosis. They need help and time to understand their disease process, and how this affects them now and in the future. However, whereas some elderly patients show a preference for letting the doctor take care of their management, most young people wish to understand what may happen next in terms of their symptoms, risks, dependency, treatment and options. This requires a degree of knowledge, experience and openness that is not always easy to find. Heart failure professionals need to have access to education for managing palliative needs and issues, support similar to their palliative colleagues and to adopt an integrated team approach.

Points to consider

- A palliative care approach and skills should be provided by the multidisciplinary and inter-agency healthcare teams involved.
- Specialist palliative care services should need to be involved only occasionally.
- Education of healthcare professionals in this area is needed.

Care pathways

The practical experience of palliative professionals, coupled with an increasingly integrated care pathway has enabled cancer services to develop a model of care which provides an efficient and economic form of service delivery to ensure optimal support and quality of life. Heart failure providers need to review such models and develop similar processes for their patients.

Structured pathways of care, using evidence-based protocols and algorithms may help the healthcare professional to follow a formatted management plan that is individualised to each person. This then must be communicated to each patient and their relatives. Following structured pathways of care, or responding to patients' questions, should highlight the need for further assessment of heart failure status and investigation when symptoms increase despite optimised drug therapy. For the younger patient this may involve, and indeed they may often expect, invasive interventions such as cardiac resynchronisation therapy (CRT),[4] an implantable cardioverter device (ICD),[5] or surgical options such as a left ventricular assist device (LVAD) or cardiac transplantation. Patients are often waiting 'to be sick enough' to have surgery, thinking that if medication is the treatment, surgery is an option saved for the future.

Younger patients tend to be more used to and comfortable with the technical 21st century. They are also more likely to use the technical world to help them seek answers for themselves. The Internet is an excellent source of information and support on their health and disease. Unfortunately, not all the information is regulated and they may access inappropriate information and biased views. Patient and carer expectations and understanding should be reviewed with each clinic visit. Healthcare beliefs and heart failure-specific knowledge should be challenged, and information offered and adapted as necessary.

Consideration for invasive intervention suggests the patient has a limited life expectancy and significant morbidity. While the healthcare professional may know this, it needs to be discussed with the patient and relatives, providing a trigger to begin discussions around supportive care and end-of-life decision making.[6] It needs to be accepted that this is a fluid discussion and people often change their views as situations change. At present we have a situation where patient under-standing and consent are routinely required for the process of implementing treatments, but not so routinely sought for withdrawing such therapies, or for managing end-of-life situations.[7] Patients and relatives should be made aware of the potential benefits and implications of such therapies. Explanation of treat-ment options should be careful and realistic, and healthcare professionals must address the patients' and relatives' expectations and avoid exaggerated claims of benefit.

Patients and relatives need support during the assessment process, and the subsequent wait for treatment. It is especially difficult for patients and relatives waiting for a cardiac transplant.[8,9] The waiting time is indefinable and dependent on the death of another person. Should an organ become available, there is little time to adjust to the idea. Some patients will become too sick to be transplanted, or die waiting. Similarly, as the need for CRT increases, the waiting lists will lengthen too; and since by definition these patients may have a life expectancy of months rather than years, some may die waiting, or not fully benefit from the intervention because of general associated deterioration. Recent initiatives within the NHS mean that patients with cancer no longer have to wait many weeks or months for investigation and/or treatment. We urgently need similar improve-ments to services for advanced heart failure, especially in the young.

There are also the patients for whom such interventions are not suitable or appropriate. Managing their feelings of rejection, denial or anger takes skill, sensitivity and time. In this process, being honest, consistent and clear, giving people time and permission to explore their fears and feelings in an open and non-threatening or personal manner, are all essential. Patients and relatives should not feel that they are dismissed with no further options, that palliative and supportive care are adjunct or 'second-best' options. Palliative and supportive care is integral to heart failure care, especially at this stage of management. The team supporting such patients should have access to support and clinical supervision to enhance and sustain such care.

Points to consider

- Tailored structured pathways of care can provide a framework for optimising patient management.
- Younger patients are more used to 'technology'.
- Younger patients are more likely to actively seek information.
- Waiting for transplantation or CRT is stressful for patient and carer.
- Patients not suitable for intervention must be handled with sensitivity.

Recognising mortality

Death is probably the last taboo in 21st-century Britain. Consequently, clear and open communication regarding prognosis and end-of-life issues is not provided for many people with heart failure, particularly the younger patient.

There is one factor common to all humans, and that is that we shall all die. How and when is unknown to most of us, and is generally not something we often contemplate. Many young people have not had exposure to death and grief. They therefore often have no experience, coping strategies or exposure to the processes and language associated with dying. Older generations frequently have some experience and understanding of death – from war experiences through to family and friends. Many older people will talk about their peers being ill and dying. There is frequently an acceptance that they have lived and nearing death, even though this may be an abstract acceptance. A lack of death or grieving experience and vocabulary may make it difficult for the younger patient to introduce the subject, and as such they may also miss the healthcare professional's probing questions.

Older people have often reached a reflective phase of their life, while very young people are in planning phases of life. Older people have experiences and memories to look back on; they have an identity and achievements to reflect on. Young people have few achievements or memories, and often have not yet established their identity. Lost time, experiences and achievements should be recognised, and permission to grieve for these may be required. Less experience means they may also have fewer coping mechanisms and less understanding of the mechanics of the healthcare system.

Young people frequently do not expect to die prematurely, even though they may know and understand their diagnosis.[10] This makes discussing the potential of sudden death particularly difficult; indeed, young people often have difficulty recognising and accepting they will die at any stage. They cannot imagine not being part of life or how to plan for their future and that of their family and friends. There is frequently a great deal of anger associated with the diagnosis and prognosis. It is difficult for family and friends to recognise and accept that this is a terminal condition and there are no cures. Young people need to recognise and accept their dying state, to plan for and gain some sense of control over their death. They may need practical help to write a will, get their affairs in order and make funeral arrangements.

Unrealistic expectations and denial can mean that family and friends find it difficult to cope with the present situation, and ignore the future changes required. This deprives the young heart failure patient of valuable and necessary support and assistance, both physical and psychosocial. Confusion and lack of clarity about the disease trajectory and prognosis is common and unsettling, and difficult to cope with, and this exacerbates the feelings of uselessness, denial and unrealistic expectation.

Points to consider

- Younger patients do not expect a premature death even if they know and understand their diagnosis.
- Younger patients may have little experience of death or little understanding of the language of dying.

Understanding heart failure

There is a general knowledge and acceptance of cancer, its treatment options and prospect of death. Many people will know of someone who has or had cancer. This is often not the case with heart failure. Its treatment and effects are generally not well understood by the general public. This can make it difficult for friends, neighbours and society to understand the needs of people with heart failure, and this in turn can lead to a feeling of frustration and isolation. The need to explain their illness and symptoms often means that people avoid discussing their heart failure with people outside their immediate family and healthcare professionals.

This may mean that young people with heart failure are more dependent on healthcare professionals for information, support and the ability to discuss their fears and concerns.[11,12] Many will wait for the professionals to raise issues around death, coping and end of life. To tackle this difficult agenda, professionals require support and training, and the confidence to become more proactive in encouraging young patients to discuss difficult issues. If patients are to accept their diagnosis and prognosis and achieve a reasonable quality of life, they and their carers will also need information and support.[10,11] There needs to be a shift in emphasis from the medical model towards a practical, psychosocial strategy, implementing more holistic care.

Physical needs

Young people will often not highlight needs because they do not wish to accept that they exist or that they are irreversible. Physical needs are often linked to medication, with symptoms being confused with side effects of drugs, or belief that the medication is not working or asking for further intervention. If the physical symptoms and altered functional needs are assessed and addressed early, many can be minimised and stabilised for longer periods, thus improving quality of life.

To ensure the appropriate information and support is delivered at the pace and level required, assessments and evaluation of needs are required at frequent intervals. The single patient assessment policy which is now proposed should ensure an initial comprehensive assessment of physical and psychosocial needs. This, however, does not obviate the need for regular follow-up, and clear and timely communication is mandatory between primary and secondary care.

Younger people have particular difficulty in accepting many physical symptoms associated with reduced functional capacity. A slower pace and being breathless when 'running' for a bus, climbing stairs or walking up a slope may be viewed as part of the ageing process and therefore tolerated as inevitable in older patients. This is not so with younger people, who may be acutely embarrassed by such signs and avoid activities which further restrict their functional capacity, which can lead to social isolation and depression.

Exercise and activity

Exercise is an essential component of physical and mental health. An inability to exercise regularly therefore impairs such health. Young people need access to advice on how to exercise, to improve their physical and mental health, and to delay the progression of heart failure and death. Access to cardiac rehabilitation programmes is rare for young people with heart failure. There are very few rehabilitation programmes specifically for heart failure, and some cardiac rehabilitation programmes will not accept heart failure referrals. People who have heart failure secondary to ischaemic heart disease may get access to rehabilitation programmes, but these are generally in older age groups.

Exercise training should be commenced on diagnosis, and young people tend to be working or studying at this point. They may not have sufficient time and energy to manage day-to-day living, and so may reduce exercise, because they link the tiredness and breathlessness associated with exercise to their disease. The benefits of exercise, together with practical guidelines on how to do it, need to be available and reiterated frequently. The NICE heart failure guidelines[3] state that patients need access to informed support on exercise, but not all clinicians have the knowledge, experience or confidence to educate their patients.

Exercise training and guidance may improve quality of life and delay functional deterioration, but must not be viewed in isolation. Access to gyms and exercise classes may be more the norm to younger generations, but young people may need to discuss practical implications such as time, cost, pacing themselves and body image first. An acceptance of their present level of fitness and function is required, with an understanding of what to expect. Setting small realistic goals in exercise training will encourage engagement and improve chances of success.

Points to consider

- Exercise training improves quality of life and delays functional deterioration.
- Younger patients may feel self-conscious about body image and so be reluctant to join a gym.

Physical support

Young patients often find it difficult to access timely physical support. Elderly people will often have their physical daily needs assessed – because of their age if not their diagnosis. There is a general assumption that young people can self-care, with the result that their daily needs are not noted in hospital or the outpatient setting. It is assumed that because you are young, you can cope without help. As we get older, we often slowly learn to adapt physically and emotionally to altering physical function, and these adaptations and coping mechanisms are often shared within our peer group. This is not the case with younger patients. Any information and advertisement regarding equipment generally features older people, making it appear less attainable and attractive to younger people.

Young people are often confused, frustrated and angry at their reduced functional ability. They may see their reduced function as a failure of the treatment, not a progression of the condition. Explaining the disease trajectory and addressing expectations may enable the individual to accept, adapt and cope better, enhancing the patient's experience, satisfaction and quality of life.

Honest and open discussion of individual physical needs encourages long-term engagement. If periodic reviews are built into heart failure management it then becomes easier to identify changes and manage these effectively. Recognising the needs is only part of the problems, however. Heart failure professionals should be aware of the services available within their community, and how to access them.

Multi-agency working

Effective care for heart failure patients of any age requires an integrated multi-agency approach: engaging, educating and supporting colleagues in a variety of settings. It requires advanced communication; an openness and willingness to share experiences and learn from and with each other; and an ability to raise the profile of heart failure and its effects on patients and their carers. Heart failure patients need access to personal and domestic care, financial and social support, irrespective of age. It is vital to avoid confusion and duplication by including all parties (patient, family, carer) and to have a designated key worker.

Eligibility for NHS-funded continuing care is reliant on individual healthcare needs assessment, not diagnosis or exact life expectancy. Patients should not be exempt because a clear life expectancy cannot be guesstimated. Not all heart failure professionals are aware of the form DS1500 (which accelerates benefit claims for ill patients), or feel confident to complete the form – what if the patient does not die within six months? Access to informed staff who are able to keep abreast of changing benefit and social care rules is an essential requirement to ensure patients are able to choose where they wish to live and die. The completion of care and benefit forms in themselves is a daunting undertaking. The forms tend to be worded in a very general way and to be badly suited to the young person with fluctuating personal, physical, mental and social needs.

> **Points to consider**
> - Young people need access to the personal and domestic care, and financial help that is so often missed.
> - Multi-agency support is required to find social and financial solutions.

Family and carers

The needs of the elderly are obvious, and accepted by other health, social services and voluntary agencies, but not so the needs of the younger heart failure patient, which are therefore frequently unmet. The burden of care frequently falls on parents, children, partners and others, who often do not identify themselves as 'carers'. A spouse or child will frequently adjust to changing circumstances within the home, adopting a variety of tasks and roles previously held by the patient. This can have a dramatic impact on relationships and the family dynamics.

The needs of carers are acknowledged in the Carers (Equal Opportunities) Act, but the practicalities involved in addressing their needs is frequently ignored or under-resourced. The 2001 Census suggests that one in 10 of the population in England and Wales are carers. Carers frequently state the ability to have a break is the most significant support they require. However, nursing home respite care may not be available or appropriate to the younger patient. Heart failure professionals need access to information regarding such available resources, and there needs to be recognition of the impact of heart failure on patients and their carers. Greater research of the daily reality of living with young people with heart failure will enhance understanding and recognition.

Young carers can experience a protracted grieving process while their loved one dies slowly of heart failure. Also, when a spouse becomes a carer, this subtly changes the balance of the relationship. The increasing physical, mental and emotional strain experienced by the carer is often not noted or acknowledged by the patient, carer, family and healthcare professionals. This can result in carer and patient unmet needs, frustrations, isolation and impaired or maladaptive coping mechanisms.

In both the short and long term, this will affect how they (carers and patients alike) cope and feel, and how they perceive and accept the diagnosis and prognosis. Time is important when the future is unsure, and emotional concerns and needs are rarely given priority over physical tasks. Accessing physical support in the form of personal care, housework or shopping can relieve the carer and give them time to engage in more positive activities such as organising a social gathering or simply enjoying a film with the patient. For many, the extended period of uncertainty in heart failure means lives are put on hold, and the emotional and physical stresses and tension are for a longer period than experienced with most types of cancer.

It can be particularly hard for parents to have an increasingly dependent child who is a young adult. It comes at a stage when their peers' children are leaving home, settling down and starting families of their own, free from childcare responsibilities. On a physical level it can be hard to go back to disturbed nights, basic hygiene care and lifting a heavy adult when no longer young themselves.

On a psychological level, it is hard to deal with the loss of the child's future, loss of potential grandchildren and loss of fulfilment of potential. There are inevitable worries about what may happen to the child should anything happen to them. For the patient, it can be hard to be cared for again by the parent, often after a period of independence, feeling as if they are a young child again, or a burden.

Points to consider

- Illness creates tensions and changes in roles within families.
- Carers become exhausted and respite care is difficult to find for the younger patient.
- A young adult being cared for by parents can cause particular strain on the parent–child relationship.

Sexual needs

Carers who physically care for a loved one engage in regular physical contact of a non-sensual or sexual nature. This may mean that physical contact is confined to such tasks. We all need to be and feel loved. A lack of personal physical contact can be distressing to all family members, but partners especially. We are sexual beings, and our sexual needs are no less important because we are ill and dying.

There are physical and emotional reasons why people with heart failure experience sexual problems. The most obvious issue is a lack of energy and functional ability. People who are used to exercising regularly and able to tolerate a degree of breathlessness through training will manage the physical concerns better. Discussing the issue and practical solutions, like resting and avoiding heavy meals prior to sexual intercourse and trying different positions, can help. Impaired cardiac output affects the blood supply to the skin and sexual organs, which can result in impaired sensation and pleasure, and ability to have or maintain an erection. Drugs can further affect this through their side effects, their effect on lowering blood pressure or on the mucous membranes (diuretics). An assessment of sexual function and need is a delicate task and not performed regularly, but can be linked to discussion of exercise, drug therapy and psychosocial wellbeing.

Sexual and sensual pleasure is not confined to penetration. Recognising and discussing needs can help to find alternative ways to provide sexual pleasure. Fears, frustrations, misunderstandings and expectations can unnecessarily restrict sexual activity. Patients and partners need to understand and accept the diagnosis and reality of life with heart failure. Fears about physical ability and risk should be sensitively explored and challenged. Practical suggestions regarding minimising exertion are important factors to easing this embarrassing subject. Positions that require supporting the body through the arms may not be realistic in many patients who have weak and cachexic arm muscles. This weakness can also inhibit masturbation. Very close intimate contact can be uncomfortable and claustrophobic to the breathless patient.

Apart from the natural fear of embarrassment, professionals may avoid raising the issue of sexual needs because of their lack of knowledge and resources for managing such issues. Access to erectile dysfunction clinics and materials, and relationship and sexual counselling should be available to heart failure teams to empower them to assess and meet such needs.

Points to consider

- Sexual contact is often important.
- Assessment can be broached in the context of psychosocial wellbeing.

Body image

Heart failure can seriously affect body image, which in turn affects self-confidence, sexuality, mood and willingness to self-care. Women with heart failure are frequently heard to lament 'the loss of the only thin part of them' as they look at their swollen ankles. Heart failure and its management can cause swollen ankles, a distended abdomen, muscle loss, thinning and dry skin, peeling lips, altered colour (including jaundice, blue lips, white/blue peripheries, red and weeping cellulitic legs, red/brown chronically engorged legs), alopecia, gynaecomastia, a dry, irritating cough and a runny nose, to mention just a few of the frustrating and inconvenient physical characteristics. Physical appearance is important to all humans, being part of our identity. Such physical characteristics and limitations (peripheral coolness, postural dizziness and urinary frequency) affect our choice of clothes, shoes, activities and social interactions. This is a major handicap for young single people who wish to interact with their peers, and seek opportunities to meet new friends and potential partners.

The need to procreate

Sexual intercourse is not simply a physical and emotional need, there is the need in all of us to procreate. The wish to have a child is universally acknowledged, but may be impossible for a young person with heart failure. Such a missed opportunity can have a significant impact on the emotional wellbeing of the patient and their partner. It leads to feelings of inadequacy, failure, frustration and depression. The need to have a child is linked to our sense of the continuity of life, and the realisation that when we die we leave nothing of ourselves behind is difficult to cope with. This can have serious affects on relationships, and is especially difficult to manage in some ethnic cultures where procreation is an essential part of marriage and identity.

Informed heart failure staff should discuss the implications and risks associated with having a child with access to associated services. Men with heart failure who wish to have a child need to explore the physical possibilities of impregnating their partner. If maintaining an erection is difficult, guidance regarding erectile aids and suitable positions that minimise effort and function for the man need to be discussed. It is important to remember that drugs such as sildenafil (Viagra) lower the blood pressure and may require several doses over time to reach optimal effect. If such physical effort or erectile function is not possible, alternative services such as IVF may be considered.

The physical effects associated with pregnancy and delivery make pregnancy for some heart failure females inadvisable. The potential effect on the mother and foetus (from drugs especially) should be sensitively and explicitly explored with both partners. In the few cases where pregnancy does occur, specialist antenatal care should be accessed immediately, and specialist postnatal care after the birth. The risks of planned or spontaneous termination should be discussed, and the risks of birth defects. Collaborating with local 'high-risk' maternity services ensures access to appropriate support, investigations and management.

It is therefore essential that the topic be raised with all heart failure patients of childbearing age, and methods of contraception discussed. There are limited choices available to women with heart failure. The thromboembolic risks associated with the contraceptive pill make this an unattractive and inadvisable method. The sheath is often not a practical option due to the other physical limitations associated with sexual intercourse for people with heart failure, and its relatively poor reliability makes it an undesirable choice where pregnancy is absolute contraindicated. Heart failure professionals may need to work with contraceptive services to offer the support and advice necessary to couples.

Such co-ordinated working is also required to address the genetic issues which patients with familial or idiopathic cardiomyopathy face. Information regarding genetic counselling, family screening and linking in to paediatric cardiac services should be available and discussed with parents and couples planning a family. Practical concerns of raising a family should be discussed, such as financial and childcare constraints. Parents need to be aware of what services and information they can access for practical parenting issues, and how to plan for the future with their children.

Points to consider

- Men may need guidance regarding erectile dysfunction.
- Women need specialist pre/ante/postnatal care it they wish to become pregnant.
- Counselling is required about the risk of birth defects and the cardiovascular risk of pregnancy.

Needs of children

Children in particular find it difficult to cope with a parent being chronically ill and dying. The needs of children may be ignored because of the professional's and patient's fears about how to handle the situation sensitively. Heart failure professionals who engage honestly in discussions about end-of-life and supportive care are likely to identify such needs. It is important to access the appropriate training and resources to cope with such complex emotional needs. Being aware of the wider healthcare team enables contact with school nurses, health visitors, professional counselling and bereavement services, social workers and paediatric services.

Not being there for their children in the future is a major concern of dying parents. These fears should be addressed and practical suggestions explored to help them cope and feel part of their child's future, such as writing letters, making tapes or videos, leaving treasured personal belongings and making plans for their education or holidays. Some parents compile photo albums, music tapes and make or buy gifts to be given to their children in the future.

The needs of children are paramount in paediatric palliative care services, and experiences and knowledge may be shared to enhance and develop heart failure palliative care services for young people. The expertise of paediatric services is especially relevant when planning palliative services for adolescent heart failure patients.

Point to consider

- Younger patients may have young children who will therefore lose a parent at a young age.

Transition

The transition from a paediatric to adult service is a developing area of cardiology, and HF services need to engage such experience, and utilise their understanding and expertise in developing service models to support this vulnerable client group. The needs of both the patient and their family require careful assessment and planning. The philosophy and expectations of paediatric and adult services vary considerably, and they are frequently separated geographically.

Many children make the transition from paediatric to adult services with a lack of co-ordination between relevant agencies, and little or no involvement from the young person or their family. There is inadequate planning and communication, which leads to despondency, frustration and potentially lost opportunities. Uniform access to integrated service provision would minimise confusion and sudden loss of support and services.

The family is a key consideration in managing children with a terminal illness. Family and personal carers do not necessarily have the same recognition or available support in young adult services.

End-of-life choices

The vision of the government's choice initiative encompasses equity and responsive care provision to individual needs, and requires resources and an empowered patient to work. The language associated with palliative and supportive care is unfamiliar to many, and can increase confusion and distress unless broached with sensitivity. The terms 'palliative care' and 'hospice' are emotive words that can adversely influence patients' acceptance of services, with many believing that hospice care involves stopping all medication and giving in to death. It is important to generate discussion around their understandings, misunderstandings, beliefs and expectations.

Discussions with patients and families about palliative and hospice care can be difficult for even the most experienced professional. Planning transition to palliative or supportive care begins with exploring and accepting the patient's and family's understanding of heart failure, prognosis, expectations, fears and wishes. Using questions that facilitate and encourage discussion of such emotional needs in a safe environment, avoiding emotive terminology, encourages acceptance of some of the issues and changes the focus from treating the disease to living and coping with the disease.

An early acceptance of the potentially terminal nature of the condition, with an understanding of the practical implications, prepares people for the future. Practical and ethical decisions taken and understood make the end-of-life period less traumatic. Access to acceptable, appropriate and realistic service provision facilitates choice in place of death for more people. It ensures clarity between all service providers and family members, preventing unrealistic expectations and demands, unwanted admissions and clinical interventions. Clear instructions about what to do and who to contact in particular situations enhance carers' sense of control and comfort. It is important that carers and families recognise their own emotional and physical needs in the dying phase. Failure to do so can make bereavement and recovery after the patient's death difficult.

Point to consider

- Sensitive communication is key to allowing patient choice with regard to end-of-life care.

Public and user involvement

Public and user involvement is currently a political driving force in healthcare provision strategy. It provides an excellent opportunity for patients and their carers to share their experiences, highlight needs and shape the future for heart failure care. The Modernisation Agency suggests that users becoming involved in the planning, delivering and evaluating of heart failure services could '… alter the culture of clinical care and emphasise elements which may be less technical but more important from the patients' perspective'.

Such involvement requires trust and recognition of the value of the patient's involvement, and is dependent on the patient having a sense of control of their heart failure management. Informed patients empowered and supported to self-care on diagnosis, with access to appropriately trained and skilled integrated multidisciplinary teams, should not need access to specialist palliative care services routinely. This should remove the uncertainty and confusion surrounding referrals, ensuring people have access to supportive and practical help when they most need it, and so are able to readily exercise their right of choice to their place of living and dying.

Conclusion

Specific evidence from randomised clinical trials may not be available for managing young people with palliative heart failure needs, but there are patients in this group needing care now. The challenge is to identify, extrapolate and reflect on available evidence, models and healthcare systems or structures, and marry these to the palliative needs of young people with heart failure. The next challenge will be to document, audit and publish such findings, and engage young people to reflect on their needs, problems encountered and possible solutions, as well as any positive aspects of care or the system. Integrated care teams that actively seek patient and family involvement, honest and open communication, and manage and reflect on expectation, will support and educate not only the patient and family, but also team members. The author hopes that this chapter will contribute towards helping a range of professionals to meet this challenge.

References

1 Lynn J, Teno JM, Phillips RS *et al.* Perceptions by the family members of the dying experience of older and seriously ill patients. *Ann Intern Med* 1997; **126**: 97–106.
2 Department of Health. Coronary Heart Disease Collaborative. Available from www.modern.nhs.uk/chd
3 National Institute for Health and Clinical Excellence. *Management of Chronic Heart Failure in Adults in Primary and Secondary Care*. NICE, London, 2003.
4 Linde C, Leclerq C, Rex S *et al.* Long-term benefits of biventricular pacing in congestive heart failure: resume from the Multislice Stimulation in Cardiomyopathy (MUSTIC) study. *J Am Coll Cardiol* 2002; **40**: 111–16.
5 Young JV, Abraham WT, Smith AL *et al.* Combined cardiac resynchronisation and implantable cardioversions defibrillation in advanced chronic heart failure: the MIRA-CLE ICD trial. *JAMA* 2003; **289**: 2685–94.
6 Berger J. The ethics of deactivating implanted cardioverter defibrillators. *Ann Intern Med* 2005; **142**: 631–4.
7 Goldstein NE, Lampert R, Bradley E, Lynn J, Krumholz HM. Management of implantable cardioverter defibrillators in end-of-life care. *Ann Intern Med* 2004; **141**: 835–8.
8 Evangelista LS, Dracup K, Moser DK *et al.* Two-year follow-up of quality of life in patients referred for heart transplant. *Heart Lung* 2005; **34**: 187–93.
9 Castle H, Jones I. A long wait: how nurses can help patients through the transplantation pathway. *Prof Nurse* 2004; **19**: 37–9.
10 Murray S, Boyd K, Kendall M *et al.* Dying of lung cancer or cardiac failure: prospective qualitative interview study of patients and their carers in the community. *BMJ* 2002; **325**: 929–32.
11 Martensson J, Karlsson J, Fridlund B. Male patients with congestive heart failure and their conception of their life situation. *J Adv Nurs* 1997; **25**(3): 579–86.
12 Martensson J, Karlsson J, Fridlund B. Female patients with congestive heart failure: how they conceive their life situation. *J Adv Nurs* 1998; **28**(6): 1216–24

Chapter 10

Palliative care services for patients with heart failure

Miriam Johnson

As the broader needs of patients with heart failure become more widely recognised (*see* Chapter 1), so further challenges arise – how best to provide the
supportive and palliative care that is so clearly needed, and how should the
specialist palliative care (SPC) services be involved? This chapter will discuss
some of the barriers to SPC involvement, and offers simple descriptions of some
UK services that have been able to extend their care to patients with heart failure.

Modern SPC services in the UK originated in the voluntary sector driven by
the vision of Dame Cicely Saunders. The vast majority of patients receiving such
care had cancer, and many of today's palliative care services are funded through
cancer charities such as Macmillan Cancer Relief and Marie Curie Cancer Care.
Palliative care professionals therefore have most experience with cancer patients
and may feel that their general medical knowledge is outdated. Conversely, as
medical management of heart failure by cardiologists becomes more and more
interventional, and 'optimum management' includes more and more options, it
seems to be difficult for cardiologists to admit that the focus of care should be
palliative. Because of difficulties in prognosis, there may be a reluctance to consider or discuss palliative care until the patient is almost moribund. Where liaisons
have developed between the two disciplines in the UK, it has tended to be where
the staff have had a particular personal interest, rather than through any systematic development of a service.

The importance of the palliative care approach, with the back-up of the specialist
team, has been highlighted in the Department of Health's National Service Framework for coronary disease, '…a palliative approach with help from palliative care
specialists can improve a patient's quality of life…'.[1]

The other main driver for progress in the area of both improving liaison between
cardiology and palliative care, and encouraging a palliative approach, has been
the deployment of heart failure specialist nurses, often funded through the British Heart Foundation – again a charitable resource.

More recently the Coronary Heart Disease (CHD) Collaborative,[2] a statutory
initiative, is encouraging supportive and palliative care for patients with heart
failure, working with clinicians and commissioners regionally to try to overcome existing barriers to care. Likewise, the National Council for Palliative Care
and Help the Hospices have become involved in collaborative working between
palliative care services and cardiology. However, progress is patchy and
hampered by historical structures and attitudes. Lack of NHS funding for service development means that extra burdens may fall on voluntary sector

organisations, which often have precarious funding and are concerned about potentially overloading the service.

Generic supportive and palliative care services

The importance of generic palliative care skills has been emphasised elsewhere in this book. Generic palliative care is that which should be provided by all healthcare workers irrespective of specialty and setting. The principles of symptom control based on a holistic assessment that includes physical, psychological and spiritual domains should be familiar to all health professionals, and should be sufficient to deal with all but the most complex issues. Increasingly, nursing staff in particular are becoming aware of patient needs in these areas, and heart failure nurse specialists, district nurses, practice nurses (who have often gained great skill in running chronic disease management clinics) and community matrons can play an important role in co-ordinating care. Sadly, however, this does not always extend to the cardiologists, who may not see this area as part of their remit or skills, even to recognise and refer on, and feel too pressurised in busy clinics to deal with anything other than the obviously cardiological medication. Most general practitioners will be involved with patients who have advanced heart failure, and have experience of palliative care, but GP skills relating to chronic heart failure may be variable.

In primary care, the Macmillan Gold Standards Framework (GSF)[3] (a standardised organisational framework of multiprofessional care developed for palliative care needs for cancer patients, but applicable also to non-cancer patients) is being used by many general practices in the UK and fosters a consistent palliative approach for patients who are likely to be in their last 6–12 months of life. Emphasis is placed on co-ordination of care, anticipatory planning and prescribing, communication (particularly with the out-of-hours services) and supporting a patient's preferred place of care if possible.

The importance of including non-cancer patients in GSF has been highlighted,[4] as 19% of deaths are due to heart disease. Analysis of data from phase 4 of the GSF project[3] showed that 67.3% of primary care teams at 12 months had already included non-cancer patients on the Supportive Care Register, although it is suspected that the threshold for inclusion is still too high. Four criteria suggested by the CHD collaborative are:

1 NYHA class III/IV
2 patient thought by care team to be in the last year of their life
3 repeated hospital admissions with heart failure symptoms
4 difficult symptoms despite optimum tolerated therapy.

Fragmentation of care is a real risk because of the increasing numbers of healthcare professionals involved in a patient's care, and GSF is a practical way of trying to find a way of working together to minimise this.

In secondary care, there is the challenge of frequent staff changeover, and the SPC team is often used greatly in educating the ward-based staff in generic palliative care skills. Prompts of care such as the Liverpool Care Pathway for the Dying[5] can enable the generic team to care well for all but the most complex cases. This is discussed more fully in Chapter 8.

Table 10.1 Services that may be useful for heart failure patients

Setting	Possible role
Hospital team	Symptom control, psychological support to patient and carer, financial and benefits advice, support and education to ward team, rationalisation of medication, help with communication issues and end-of-life decisions, Liverpool Care Pathway, outpatient clinic with palliative physician
Community team	As above but in patient's own home, education and support of primary care team, palliative consultant domiciliary visit/ phone advice, hospice at home
Hospice team	*Inpatient admission* for appropriate patients: symptom control, fluid balance and optimisation of diuretic therapy, psychological and spiritual support, end-of-life care, carer support and bereavement care
	Day hospice attendance for social isolation, regular symptom monitoring with weight and diuretic balance, physiotherapy and occupational therapy review
	Out-of-hours palliative care telephone advice and support
	Outpatient clinic with palliative physician

Specialist palliative care services

SPC services span the boundaries of hospital, community and hospice, and are multiprofessional. Doctors and nurse specialists are the usual core members of the team, but many teams also have physiotherapists, occupational therapists, pharmacists, chaplains and social workers. Therefore there are many services that may be useful for heart failure patients (Table 10.1).

The model of involvement will of necessity vary from place to place, for example the service in a district general setting will be different to that in a busy city teaching hospital. In a district setting, the same palliative physician may be involved in hospital, hospice and community, whereas in a city there are likely to be separate teams.

Barriers to involving SPC services

There are three main common concerns: that SPC services will be overwhelmed, that heart failure patients would not want to be referred to SPC services and that SPC services could not provide appropriate care for heart failure patients.

Palliative care services will be overwhelmed

There are concerns that SPC services will be overwhelmed by the demand,[6,7] and precious beds in short-stay acute units will become blocked by patients with severe debility, but not imminently dying. The less well-defined terminal phase in heart failure adds to this fear. Even where it is acknowledged that numbers may not be overwhelming, there are concerns that this group of patients may make a comparatively high demand on the service.[7] However, referral to special-ist palliative care services should only be necessary in patients with difficult symptoms or psychosocial issues, with the majority being well cared for by their cardiologist and general practitioner.[8] As practices adapt and adopt the Macmillan GSF for palliative care in primary care, so a co-ordinated and anticipatory approach should improve the standard of care for these patients. Likewise, in the community or hospital, the Liverpool Care Pathway for the Dying has improved the standard of care without requiring the specialist team to be directly involved. Therefore the numbers of patients who require the specialist services may not be as great as feared. Experience from the St George's Project,[9] the Bradford experience and from Scarborough[10] would suggest that approximately 10% of patients with heart failure known to the heart failure nurse specialist will require access to one of the SPC services.

Patients would not want referral to a hospice

Other concerns have centred on the acceptability of 'hospice' or 'palliative care' to patients with heart failure. Understandably it is hard for cardiologists or gen-eral practitioners to introduce this into a discussion, and there will be some heart failure patients (as there are cancer patients) who cannot cope with the idea of being referred. However, with good communication skills, this should not be a major problem for the majority. Patient satisfaction questionnaires from 22 heart failure patients referred to the hospital palliative care team in Torbay showed that all patients found contact with the SPC team acceptable. Using a multiprofessional approach across primary and secondary care, workload was manageable within available resources.[11] Likewise, the service provided by Paul Paes[12] was deemed highly satisfactory by patients. The heart failure nurse specialist is likely to be a helpful liaison point in this regard.

Palliative care staff do not have the necessary skills

Will hospice staff be able to manage patients admitted for heart failure? The majority of interventions should be well within the field of specialist palliative care skills, with only a few 'new' skills (patient weighing, fluid balance and intravenous diuretics) to be learned if admissions for decompensation as well as end-of-life care are to be available. Mutual support and education between car-diology and the hospice will be needed for this to happen. In a hospital-based questionnaire,[13] Dharmasena and Forbes reported that if there was a palliative care service extended to non-malignant patients, then 94% of responding phy-sicians would consider referring their patients to it. It was considered that the most appropriate form of service should be one of shared care and responsibility, which would address concerns regarding lack of disease-specific skills in the palliative care team.

Progress so far

Palliative care service provision for heart failure patients is patchy in the UK.

Gibbs[14] surveyed over 400 UK SPC services in 2004 to see what services, education and training were provided. Of the 200 responses (43% response rate) only one service stated there was no role for SPC in heart failure and only four services would not accept patients with heart failure. However, patient numbers were low, with most having only 0–3 current patients under their care. Seven services had 4–11 patients; one had 18. An active partnership seemed to be the most successful model with the heart failure nurse specialist remaining as 'key worker'. Regular support, education and communication with the SPC services were important. The SPC services would provide advice, short-term intervention or 'full' SPC for as few patients as appropriate. Specific guidelines, including triggers to assist identification of patients who are appropriate for consideration of SPC referral, were important and adopting the GSF definition ('sick enough that dying in the next year would not be a surprise') had been found to be helpful.

Examples of palliative care services involved with heart failure patients

Although engagement of SPC services in heart failure has been relatively cautious, some centres are developing along these lines. We include summary descriptions here by way of encouragement, and to give a reference source to any interested professionals. They are not meant to be definitive models by any means, but merely examples of relatively established initiatives that appear to be working in their respective localities. Each description is provided by the professionals involved.

Bradford

(Contributed by Andrew Daley, Marie Curie Hospice, Maudsley Street, Leeds Road Bradford BD3 9LH)

In 2002, three of the Bradford primary care trusts (PCTs) each appointed a heart failure nurse specialist. The nurses formed a team, whose aim was to support people at home following a hospital admission for heart failure.

None of the nurses appointed had specialist palliative care experience. However, they decided from the outset that providing (or facilitating) good supportive and palliative care was an important part of their role. They made early links with the local SPC services, attending their multidisciplinary meetings to learn informally from the teams' case discussions and to have the opportunity of discussing some of their own cases. The services also collaborated educationally, delivering joint sessions for primary care teams and organising formal events at which palliative care and heart failure staff could learn from each other.

One of the palliative care consultants has been involved with the heart failure nurse specialist team from its outset, being part of the multidisciplinary steering group driving service developments and championing the collaboration of the heart failure nurse specialist and SPC services at a local and national level.

In 2003, the PCTs agreed a modest increase in funding for day centre places for non-cancer patients at the Marie Curie hospice. A big Lottery bid for a psychologist to work with non-cancer patients was also successful. These developments allowed the establishment of a support group for people with heart failure and their carers. The group is run weekly by the heart failure nurse specialist team in the hospice day centre and scores highly on evaluations. It provides:

- social interaction and informal emotional support in a comfortable, non-clinical environment
- group relaxation and breathing training
- 1:1 professional support as necessary – by palliative care nurses, heart failure nurses, psychologist, dietician, benefits advisor, physiotherapist or palliative care physician
- a rolling programme of structured sessions covering drugs, nutrition, exercise, psychological wellbeing and benefits advice.

It has become clear that the heart failure nurse specialist team is itself capable of co-ordinating excellent care until death for the majority of people. Additional support often takes the form of telephone advice from a palliative care consultant or Macmillan nurse. So far, direct involvement of the SPC services has been required or less than 20% of their patients.

- Support group attendance   10%
- Medical outpatient assessment   4%
- Standard hospice day therapy attendance   4%
- Hospice at home nursing   3%
- Joint home visit with Macmillan nurse   2%
- Hospice inpatient care   1%

Our experience demonstrates that high-quality palliative care can be provided by heart failure nurse specialists with support from the existing SPC services. This support can be provided at a modest cost in terms of time and resources.

Scarborough[10]

(Contributed by Miriam Johnson, St Catherine's Hospice, Throxenby Lane, Scarborough YO12 5RE)

In 2001, one of the consultant palliative physicians and the cardiologist from the district general hospital (population 230,000) set up a shared-care approach for heart failure patients. As in Bradford, the palliative physician has been involved in the PCT's coronary heart disease group, and this worked well with the successful bid to the British Heart Foundation for heart failure nurse specialists, three of whom were appointed in 2004. Unlike Bradford, the services developed prior to heart failure nurse specialist appointment, but have been strengthened further since, with the SPC staff (particularly the nurses) feeling supported by them. Referral criteria are agreed between cardiology and palliative care.
    Services available for heart failure patients are as follows.

- Hospital inpatients can be assessed by consultant palliative physician and have access to the hospital palliative care nurse specialist. In addition, the Liverpool Care Pathway for the Dying is in use throughout, which means that the specialist team is often not required for patients requiring straightforward terminal care.

- The consultant palliative physician has outpatient clinics both in the hospital and in the hospice. Patients can access these according to preference.
- The day hospice provides access to weekly multiprofessional review as required. Patients become familiar with hospice surroundings and staff, and in practice, many of these patients have opted for hospice admission rather than hospital, should admission become necessary.
- Hospice admission is an option for patients who require symptom control or terminal care. Intravenous diuretics and daily fluid balance with weighing can be provided for appropriate patients – facilitated by easy access to cardiology support. A review of admissions since the beginning of the service in March 2005 showed that, in the main, the care given was well within the skills of specialist palliative care.[10] The only main culture change was weighing patients – rarely used in palliative oncology. The willingness of the hospice to take patients for intravenous diuretics even if it is not clear that the patient is dying, may be the reason why the number of hospital deaths is reducing in favour of home or hospice according to patient choice.
- Domiciliary assessment by, and telephone advice from, a consultant palliative physician can be accessed by general practitioners.
- The heart failure nurse specialists often attend practice GSF meetings, which appears to be improving anticipatory care for these patients.
- Advanced communication skills training. The hospice education department runs the Maguire-Faulkner communications skills course and consultant cardiologists and heart failure nurse specialists have now been trained.

The demand on the service is slowly increasing, now averaging 20–30 referrals a year, which is approximately 10% of the patients known to the heart failure nurse specialists. It is a relatively small percentage of the specialist palliative care team work load, although enough to maintain skills.

Merseyside & Cheshire Palliative Care Network

(Contributed by Clare Littlewood, Palliative Care Team, Whiston Hospital, Warrington Road, Prescot, Liverpool L35 5DR)

Merseyside & Cheshire has a well-established palliative care network. To avoid duplication throughout the network, a subgroup for non-malignant disease was formed in 2002, with the aim of developing network-wide symptom control, referral guidelines and service directory for non-malignant diseases. Advanced heart failure was the first chronic disease to be looked at. Guidelines were developed and distributed both locally and nationally.[15]

A complex heart failure clinic has been developed at Whiston hospital using a collaborative model of care. A palliative medicine consultant, cardiology associate specialist and heart failure nurse specialist consult together in the monthly clinic for four to six patients, pre-selected by the heart failure nurse specialist. The cardiologist leads, concentrating on physical problems, and instigates investigations and a management plan. The palliative care physician will then address psychosocial and unresolved symptom control issues. Referral to day hospice and other agencies is instigated if necessary. Leaflets about the local hospice are given to patients who are wary about coming. This has resulted in increasing numbers of referrals to all areas of specialist palliative care, not just to day therapy. It has also improved communication and education between the different professionals.

Heart failure patients are incorporated into routine day therapy with cancer patients, usually for a programme of eight weeks.

The appointment of a clinical nurse specialist in palliative care specifically for heart failure patients will further expand the service. A rehabilitation programme for advanced heart failure patients is being developed, with a session on palliative care issues being introduced. Both these developments are to be evaluated.

Torbay[8]

(Contributed by Jo Sykes and Tim Chester, Torbay Hospital, South Devon Healthcare Trust, Torquay, Devon)

Torbay Hospital is a district general hospital serving a resident population of some 250,000 across south Devon, although the numbers are swelled seasonally by the many tourists. South Devon has an integrated specialist palliative care service consisting of hospital and community teams and a hospice situated 1.5 miles from the acute hospital.

The link between the cardiology department and the hospital specialist palliative care nurses in Torbay was strengthened by the appointment of a heart failure nurse specialist and a hospital-based consultant in palliative medicine with an interest in non-malignant palliative care in 1999. Representatives from both teams agreed a set of specific guidelines to encourage referral to the palliative care team. A referral pathway was also produced to show how referrals would be dealt with, and that patients may be discharged back to the cardiology team if appropriate. We set out to conduct the service within the normal workings of both teams and using existing resources.

Twelve patients were referred during the first year and 10 during the second. Satisfaction questionnaires to elicit the acceptability of this type of care to patients was prospectively collected and presented to both cardiology and palliative care teams to keep the profile of the project high. The results showed that patients were being referred based on need rather than stage of illness, although the majority of patients had NYHA class IV heart failure. Patients were seen in the consultant outpatient clinic, on the wards and on two occasions in their own homes. Patients had a significant symptom burden, some of which was under-recognised and under-treated. Interventions included pain and symptom management and referral to other agencies such as social services, occupational therapy, physiotherapy, primary care nurses and hospice day care. All those able to be asked were satisfied with their care and no patients refused referral to specialist palliative care.

An example of a patient comment:

> 'I was pleased how quickly you responded to the referral from my cardiologist and pleased at the length of time you were prepared to sit and listen to my problems and work out solutions. The "follow-up" from the district nurse was also very prompt.'

For the majority of patients, their care remained shared between the cardiology and palliative care teams. This model would seem to offer optimal care to patients, build up trust between the teams and also lead to the further development of working relationships. The setting-up of this project has led to other initiatives that aim to improve care for this group of patients. Along with presentation of the data at various hospital meetings, a local study day attracting staff from all care settings was well attended and evaluated. Strong links between the teams has allowed us to introduce the Liverpool Care Pathway for the Dying on to the cardiology ward and thus improve generic palliative care on this ward. The heart failure nurse specialist was integral to the success and ongoing nature of this project. He has since undertaken a Diploma in Palliative Care to improve his own generic palliative care skills.

This approach to encourage and handle referrals has led to a manageable workload and would appear to reassure those worried about 'opening the flood gates'. However, it is likely that there are other eligible patients who may not have been referred to the service. Future challenges include continued evaluation of the guidelines to encourage referral of appropriate patients, and continued education in generic palliative care for those caring for this and other patient groups such as those with chronic respiratory disease.

Greenock

(Contributed by Dorothy McElroy, Ardgowan Hospice, Nelson Street, Greenock, Strathclyde PA15 1TS)

Help the Hospices offered the opportunity to apply for St James' Place Foundation funding in 2004, and a proposal to offer symptom management and psychological support for progressive heart failure patients was developed by Ardgowan Hospice in consultation with the heart failure nurse specialist and cardiologist at Inverclyde Royal Hospital.

As a patient-led cancer support drop-in centre (Living with cancer at ACCESS at Ardgowan) was already working well, it was considered suitable to extend this non-traditional model of palliative care to cardiac patients.

A programme of education for hospice staff was devised in conjunction with the heart failure nurse specialist and referral criteria were drawn up. The pilot project began to receive patients and carer referrals in April 2005. As with cancer patients attending ACCESS, the focus is on care and support in a non-clinical environment, with the locus of control being with the patient or carer.

In the first six months of the pilot, 23 patients and four carers have received support to address social isolation, anxiety, fatigue, breathlessness, fear, depression and insomnia. Support is provided through individual consultation and assessment with a nurse specialist, followed by the offer of a series of complementary therapies, relaxation sessions, modified Tai Chi and breathlessness management. Home visits may be undertaken by therapists, allowing carers to attend ACCESS for their own support.

Initially, members of staff were concerned about the potential increase in referrals and also about their own level of expertise. Good communication in relation to the project aims and information/education sessions have allayed general fears.

Future funding has yet to be secured for the continuation of the pilot; however, there is now an air of excitement within Ardgowan Hospice staff and trustees regarding this initiative and we look forward to formal evaluation of the project by staff at Southampton University.

Conclusions

Extension of specialist palliative care services to heart failure patients is in its infancy, but as the examples illustrate, it can be accomplished successfully. The fears of professionals and patients can be overcome if the specialist nurses and doctors involved take an active role in setting up a collaborative service. However, at the present time an optimum service model is not known. Until recently, there has been little engagement of or by the voluntary sector (the majority of hospices) in strategic planning of health services. SPC services have therefore grown up in a haphazard way, often at the instigation of local benefactors rather than in response to a systematic needs assessment. In the palliative care of oncology, this has changed due to the advent of cancer networks, which have embraced the need for equitable SPC services. Such an approach needs to be mirrored for patients with non-malignant disease (*see* Chapter 1), and services currently running should evaluate the acceptability and outcomes of their service.

References

1 Department of Health. National Service Framework for Coronary Heart Disease. Available from www.doh.gov.uk/nsf/coronary.htm
2 Department of Health. Coronary Heart Disease Collaborative. Available from www.modern.nhs.uk/chd
3 Department of Health. www.goldstandardsframework.nhs.uk
4 Free A. Extending the GSF to non-cancer patients. July 2005. Link from www.goldsandardsframework.nhs.uk/non_cancer.php
5 Liverpool Care Pathway for the Dying. www.lcp-mariecurie.org.uk
6 Gannon C. Palliative care in terminal cardiac failure; hospices cannot fulfil such a vast and diverse role. *BMJ* 1995; **310**: 310–11.
7 Beattie JM, Murray RG, Brittle J, Catanheira T. Palliative care in terminal cardiac failure. Small numbers of patients with terminal cardiac failure may make considerable demands on services. [Letter; comment] *BMJ* 1995; **310**: 1411.
8 Seamark DA, Ryan M, Smallwood N, Gilbert J. Deaths from heart failure in general practice: implications for palliative care. *Pall Med* 2002; **16**: 495–8.
9 Davidson PM, Paull G, Introna K, Cockburn J, Davis JM, Rees D, Gorman D, Magann L, Lafferty M, Dracup K. Integrated, collaborative palliative care in heart failure: the St. George Heart Failure Service experience 1999-2002. *J Cardiovasc Nurs* 2004; **19**: 68–75.
10 Johnson MJ, Houghton T. Palliative care for patients with heart failure – description of a service. *Pall Med* 2006; **20**: 211–14.
11 Sykes J, Chester T. Palliative care for chronic heart failure patients. [Abstract from British Cardiac Society Annual Scientific Conference, Glasgow 2003] *Heart* 2003; **89**(Suppl 1): A8(018).
12 Paes P. A pilot study to assess the effectiveness of a palliative care clinic in improving the quality of life for patients with severe heart failure. [Letter] *Pall Med* 2005; **19**(6): 505–6.
13 Dharmasena HP, Forbes K. Palliative care for patients with non-malignant disease: will hospital physicians refer? *Pall Med* 2001; **15**: 412–81.
14 Gibbs LM, Khatri AK, Gibbs JS. Survey of Specialist Palliative Care and Heart Failure: September 2004. *Palliative Medicine*. 2006, in press.
15 Cheshire and Merseyside Cardiac Network; www.cmcn.nhs.uk

Index

Page numbers in italic refer to tables.

ACE inhibitors 35
activities of daily living 79–80
acute decompensation 38–40, *38*
  see also advanced heart failure
adolescents 131
adrenaline 39–40
adrenergic innervation 24
advanced directives 100, 104
advanced heart failure
  aetiology and physiology 20–8, *38*, 46
  classification systems *11*
  co-morbidity 9–10, *10*, 46–8
  comparisons with cancer 4–9, *5–6, 7, 8–9*, 74–5
  illness trajectories 4–6, *5–6*
  language and terminology 90, 97–8, 101
  mortality studies 12, *12*, 54
  non-pharmacological therapies 40–1, *41*, 62–3, 68–9
  pharmacological therapies 31–40, *35*, 61–2, 64–70
  prevalence studies 11–12, *14*
  prognosis 7–9, *8–9*, 44–57, 91, 102–3, 104–5, 120
  psychological factors 27–8, 47, 77–8, 90
  quality of life surveys 3–4, 80
  services 42, 75, 84
  studies of patient experiences 1–2, 75–84
  symptoms 2–4, *3*, 26–8, 60–70, *63*
  young peoples needs 119–33
adverse remodelling processes 23
aetiology 20, 46
  physiological responses 20–8
  socioeconomic factors 13–15
afterload, treatment principles 21
age factors
  and aetiology 20, *21*
  and prognosis 45
  see also young people with heart failure
ageism 81
AIRE data 12, *12*
aldosterone antagonists 32
anaemia 27, 47, 65–6
analgesic ladder 66, *67*

Anderson, H *et al. 7*, 13, 61
anger 102, 126
angina 68–9
  incidence 61
angiotensin II receptor blocking agents 34
angiotensin-converting enzyme (ACE) inhibitors 35
anorexia 69
anticoagulant therapies 37
antidepressants *63*, 65
anxiety 78–9
  panic attacks 65
apnoeic breathing patterns 26, 49, 65
apoptosis of heart muscle 22
Ardgowan Hospice (Strathclyde) 142
arrhythmia 25
aspirin 37–8
assessment of need
  demographic approaches 13
  epidemiological approaches 11–13, *12*
  socioeconomic approaches 15
  young people 124–32
  see also care pathways
atrial fibrillation 25
ATLAS trial 12, *12*
atrial fibrillation 48

B-type natriuretic peptide (BNP) markers 52
beliefs and values, end-of-life issues 100
benefits and allowances 77, 79–80, 126
benzodiazepines 65
beta-adrenergic blocking agents 36, 38–9
bisoprolol 36
biventricular pacing 25, 40
blood pressure indicators 48
BMI indicators 48–9
body image 129
Bradford palliative care services 138–9
breaking bad news 93–6, 102–3
  and hope 89
breathlessness
  contributing factors 26
  management 62–5, *63*
  and prognosis 49

types 26
Buetow, S et al. 2, 76–7
bumetanide 31–2
BUN/creatinine/uric acid markers 51

CABG (coronary artery bypass graft)
    surgery 69
cachexia 48, 69
Calgary–Cambridge model 91–2
cancer co-morbidity 47
cancer–heart failure comparisons
    illness trajectories 5–6
    prognosis 7–9, 8
    support measures 74–5
    symptoms 6–7, 7
candida 69–70
cardiac cachexia 48, 69
cardiac pain 68–9
cardiac perfusion 24
cardiac resynchronisation therapy (CVT)
    25, 40
cardiac transplants 40, 41–2, 122–3
'cardio-renal' syndrome 48, 49
cardiologists 135
cardiopulmonary resuscitation (CPR) 103–
    4
    see also DNR (do not resuscitate) orders
care pathways 104, 112, 114–16
    for young people 121–3
    see also palliative care; supportive care
carers
    availability 111
    financial cost 'savings' 111
    lack of support 81
    needs assessment studies 13
    support measures 116
carvedilol 36
cellulitis 70
certification of death 12
Charlson Index 46
CHARM study (Pocock et al.) 34, 45
CHART study (Watanabe et al.) 55–6
Cheyne-Stokes breathing 26, 49
children 130–1
Christakis, NA 88
citalopram 63, 65
classification systems 11
Clausen, H et al. 81
clinical trials 119–20
clinics see heart failure clinics
co-codamol regimes 67
co-morbidity 10, 46–8
cognitive impairment 28, 47

colchicine 68
communication
    areas and scope 88
    barriers 89–93, 93
    benefits 87–8
    breaking bad news 93–6, 102–3
    end-of-life issues 77, 98–100, 102–5, 123–
        4
    lessons from oncology 93–6
    in outpatient clinics and hospitals 83, 90,
        92–3, 99–100
    over disability 82
    as 'process' 94, 96, 101
    of prognosis 77, 79, 91, 100, 101, 102–3,
        104–5
    training workshops 96–7
    within service frameworks 98
Connolly, M 99–100
constipation 69
contraception 130
coping skills 76–7, 98–9
    dealing with prognosis 88–9, 90–1, 94–6
coronary artery bypass graft (CABG)
    surgery 69
Coronary Heart Disease Collaborative 134
    support guidelines 74
cough, and ACE inhibitors 34
CPR (cardiopulmonary resuscitation) 103–
    4
    see also DNR (do not resuscitate) orders
creatinine levels 34
CRT (cardiac resynchronisation therapy)
    25, 40
cystatin C marker 51
cytokines 25–6, 69

daily activity level measurements 50
daily living activities 79–80
Davies, MK et al. 14
death certification 12
death and dying see end-of-life issues
decision-making
    models 91–2
    shared objectives 76, 87, 91–2, 98–100
demographic studies 13
denial responses 102, 124
    avoiding 'bad news' 89
depression 27–8, 47, 77–8, 90
    physiological causes 27–8, 77
    suicidal feelings 82
    treatments 63, 65, 78
device therapies see ICDs (implantable
    cardioverter devices)

diabetes 46
Dias, L *et al.* 87
digoxin 37
dihydrocodeine 64
DIPEx (Database of Individual Patient
    Experiences) 2, 76
disease trajectories 4–6, *5–6*
    and uncertainty 44, 79, 100, 102–3, 120
diuretics 31–3
    intravenous 39, 42
    and overdiuresis 32
    resistance 49
DNR (do not resuscitate) orders 100
    and ICD deactivations 103, 113–14, 115
domperidone 69
driving restrictions, opioid use 67
drug treatments 31–40, *35*, 61–2, 64–70
    joint decision-making 76
    symptom management 61–2, *63*, 64–70
dry mouth 69–70

ECG measurements 50
echocardiograph measurements 50–1
Edinburgh study (Murray *et al.*) 2, 7, 9, 61,
    74–5, 79, 82–4, 89
educational status 76
EFFECT (Enhanced Feedback for Effective
    Cardiac Treatment) study 53–4, *53*
Ellershaw, J and Ward, C 104
end-of-life issues 83–4
    care of family 116, 127–8, 130–1
    care pathways 104, 112, 114–16
    communication needs 77, 98–100, 102–5,
        123–4
    home palliative care 110–12
    hospice care 112
    hospital care 111–12
    ICD deactivations 103, 113–14, 115
    joint decision-making 76, 87, 91–2, 98–
        100
    medication adjustments 115–16
    recognition of dying phase 113–14, 115
    treatment withdrawal requests 113–14,
        115
    for young people 123–4, 131–2
enoximone 39–40
EPHesus study 32
EPICAL study (Alla *et al.*) 55, *56*
epidemiological studies 11–13, *12*
eplerenone 32
erectile dysfunction 129
ergoreflexes 26
etanercept 26

ethnicity issues 13
euphemisms 98
European Society of Cardiology 39
evidence-based care 119–20
exercise capacity 49
exercise programmes 66, 125

fatigue *63*, 65–6, *66*
financial support, benefits and allowances
    77, 79–80, 126
Formiga, F *et al.* 89
Framingham study (Kalon *et al.*) 46
Fried, TR 89
functional indicators 48–9
funding care 111, 112, 134–5
    see also benefits and allowances
furosemide 31–2

gender
    and incidence *21*
    and prognosis 46
general practitioners 84
    attitudes 81, 82, 84
genetic counselling 130
Gibbs, L 16
Gold Standard Frameworks (GSFs) 111,
    112, 135
Goldacre, MJ *et al.* 12
Goldstein, NE *et al.* 103
gout 68
Greenock palliative care services 142

haloperidol *63*, 69
Hanratty, B *et al.* 16, 93, 104–5
health services 42
    care shortfalls 75, 92–3
    funding 81, 111, 112, 134–5
    system failures 84
    team care 15
    user involvement 132
    see also palliative care
heart
    basic 'pump' model 20–2
    cell necrosis/apoptosis 22–3
    decompensation 24–5
    hormones 22
    perfusion 24
    remodelling processes 23
    renin-angiotensin-aldosterone system
        (RAAS) 23–4, *23*, 25
    rhythm and synchrony 25
    and skeletal muscle function 25–6
    sympathetic nervous system 24

Heart of England Screening Study *14*
heart failure
   causes 20, 46
   classification systems *11*
   illness trajectories 4–6, *5–6*
   incidence *21*
   natural history 38
   prognosis and indicators 7–9, *8–9*, 44–57
   see also advanced heart failure
heart failure clinics 7, 42
Heart Improvement Project 74
heart rate measurements 50
Herrmann-Lingen, C *et al.* 78
Hillingdon Study (Cowie *et al.*) 9, 45
Hinton, JM 1
Hippocrates 88
history taking 99
Hobbs, FD *et al.* 3, *3*
home adaptations 80
home palliative care 110–11
hope and uncertainty 77, 79, 89
hospice care 112, 136–43, *136*
   see also specialist palliative care services
hospital admissions
   communication problems 45, 83
   end-of-life care 111–12, *136*
   and social support 80
hydralazine 34
hypertension 48
hypertrophy 22

ICDs (implantable cardioverter devices)
   25, 40–1, *41*
   deactivation issues 103, 113–14, 115
   NICE guidance *41*
   types 40–1
illness trajectories *see* disease trajectories
implantable defibrillators *see* ICDs
   (implantable cardioverter devices)
infarction 22
infliximab 26
inotropic support 39–40
isosorbide nitrate 34, 38
itching skin 70

jargon 101
Jiang, W *et al.* 78
joint decision-making 76, 87, 91–2, 98–100
   models 91–2

Kaye, P 92, *102*
Kendall, M *et al.* 2
Kennelly, C and Bowling, A 101

language and terminology 90, 97–8, 101
laxatives *63*, 69
left ventricular assist devices (LVADs) 40–1
left ventricular failure 21
   non-pharmacological therapies 40–1
   pharmacological therapies 33–5, *35*, 37
Liverpool Care Pathway for dying patients
   104, 112, 114–16
living wills 100, 104
Löfmark, R and Nilstun, T 99
loop diuretics 31–3
lorazepam 65, 79
lormetazepam 65, 79
LVSF (left ventricular systolic ejection
   fraction) indicators 51

McCarthy, M and Addington-Hall, J 89
McKinley, RK *et al.* 6
Macmillan Gold Standard Frameworks
   (GSFs) 111, 112, 135
Maguire communication training 96
Marie Curie Hospice (Bradford) 138–9
marital status 80
   effect of caring role 127
markers for heart failure 51–2
medical jargon 101
Merseyside & Cheshire Palliative Care
   Network 140–1
metaphor use 98
metoclopramide *63*, 69
metolazone 40
metoprolol 36
Mills, M *et al.* 111–12
Minnesota Living with Heart Failure
   questionnaire 53
mirtazapine *63*, 65, 78
mood disorders 27–8
morbidity records
   use in co-morbidity studies 9–10
   use in prognosis studies 7
morphine 64, 67, 68
mortality studies 12, *54*
   mode and place of death 12–13, *12*
mouth problems 69–70
multidisciplinary care 15, 111, 114–17, 126–
   7
Murray, SA *et al.* 2, 7, 9, 61, 74–5, 79, 81–4,
   89

National Service Frameworks (NSFs), for
   Cardiovascular Disease 15, 39, 41, 134
natriuretic peptides 22, 78
nausea *63*, 69

necrosis of heart muscle 22
New York Heart Association (NYHA),
    classification systems *11*, 52
NICE guidelines 15
    on exercise regimes 125
    on implantable cardioverter
        defibrillators *41*
    on supportive care 74
nocturnal breathing patterns 26, 49, 65
noradrenaline 39–40
NSAIDs (non-steroidal anti-
    inflammatories) *63*, 67–8
nursing home care 79
nutrition, and anaemia 27

occupational therapy 80, 82
oedema
    pulmonary 21, 25
    skin problems *63*, 70
Olmsted County study (Senni *et al.*) 45
open-access heart failure clinics 42
opioids
    angina 68
    breathlessness *63*, 64
    non-cardiac pain 67
oral hygiene 112
oral thrush 69–70
orthopnoea 26, 65, *66*
osteoarthritis 46
outpatient appointments 90, 92–3
oxygen therapies 39, 42
    and breathlessness 64–5
    efficacy 65

pain 3
    cardiac 68–9
    non-cardiac 66–8
    WHO analgesic ladder *67*
palliative care 16, 42, 104–5, 135
    background attitudes 16
    communication issues 99–100, 102–5
    early studies 1
    education roles 16
    initiating interventions 44, 120, 138
    literature 1
    treatments 42
    see also specialist palliative care services;
        supportive care
panic attacks 65
Pantilat, SZ and Steimle, AE 103, 104
paracetamol regimes *63*
paroxysmal nocturnal dyspnoea 26, 65, *66*
patient coping skills 76–7, 98–100

avoiding 'bad news' 89
    dealing with prognosis 88–9, 90–1, 94–6
patient decision-making 76, 87, 91–2, 98–
    100
peak exercise cardiac power output 50
peak O$_2$ uptake 49–50
peripheral oedema, skin problems 70
pharmacological therapies *see* drug
    treatments
phosphodiesterase inhibitors 39–40
physiological testing 49–51
pregnancy 129–30
preload, treatment principles 21
prevalence studies, UK studies 11–12, *14*
primary care initiatives 111, 135, *136*
pro-atrial natriuretic peptide (Pro-ANP)
    22, 78
professionals
    attitudes to death 111–12, 114, 120
    attitudes towards communication 89,
        91–2
    distancing tactics 112
prognosis 7–9, *8–9*, 102–3
    communication issues 77, 79, 91, 99–100,
        101, 102–3, 104–5
    co-morbidity studies 46–8
    evidence base studies 44–5
    functional indicators 48–9
    general indicators 45–6
    palliative care initiation question 44, 120
    patient coping strategies 76–7, 88–9, 90–
        1, 94–6, 98–9
    physiological measurements 49–51
    scoring systems 52–6, *53–6*
    specific markers 51–2
    and uncertainty 44, 79, 100, 102–3, 104–
        5, 120
pruritus 70
psychological factors 27–8, 75–9
    anxiety 78–9
    coping skills 76–7, 88–9, 90–1, 94–5, 96,
        98–9
    dealing with uncertainty 77, 79, 91, 101,
        102–3
    depression 27–8, 47, 77–8, 90
public involvement 132
pulmonary disease 47
pulmonary oedema 21, 25

quality of life
    social problems 79–81
    spiritual problems 83–4
    surveys 3–4, 80

tools and questionnaires 53

RAAS (renin-angiotensin-aldosterone
  system) 23–4, *23*, 25
RALES study 32
RCGP, prevalence studies *14*
religious beliefs 82
remodelling processes 23
renal impairment 48
renin-angiotensin-aldosterone system
  (RAAS) 23–4, *23*, 25
research 119–20
resilience 76–7
respiratory infections 47
resynchronisation therapy 25, 40
right ventricular failure 21
risk information 100
Rogers, A *et al.* 2–3

St Catherine's Hospice (Scarborough) 139–
  40
Scarborough palliative care services 139–40
scoring systems 52–6, *53–6*
serotonin 27
service organisation 42
  care shortfalls 75, 92–3
  funding 81, 111, 112, 134–5
  health vs. social needs funding 81
  system failures 84
  user involvement 132
  see also palliative care; specialist
    palliative care services; supportive
    care
setraline *63*
sexuality 123–9
sildenafil 129
Silverberg, DS *et al.* 65–6
skeletal muscle function 25, 66
  role of cytokines 25–6
skin problems *63*, 70
sleep
  breathing patterns 26
  disturbances 27, 65, *66*
sleep apnoea 26, 49, 65
social isolation 81
social services 81
  housing adaptations 80
socioeconomic factors 13–15
sodium markers 51
specialist nurses 42, 138, 139, 140–1
specialist palliative care services 113, 136–
  8, *136*
  barriers to involvement 136–7

national examples 138–42
referral criteria 112, 136–7, 138
roles 16, 137–8
scope of practice 16, 137–8, 138–42
see also palliative care; supportive care
spinal cord stimulation 68–9
spiritual problems 81–4
  end-of-life issues 83–4
spironolactone 32
SSRIs (selective serotonin uptake
  inhibitors) *63*, 65, 78
Starling's Law 21
Stewart, S *et al.* 7
suicidal feelings 82
supplemental oxygen therapies 39, 42
SUPPORT study (Levenson *et al.*) 3–4, 44,
  115
supportive care
  defined 74
  guidelines 74–5
  for psychological problems 75–7
  for social problems 79–81
  for spiritual problems 81–4
  system failures 84
  see also palliative care; specialist
    palliative care services
'surprise' prognostic question 44, 120
survival rates
  cancers *8–9*
  heart failure 7–9, *8–9*
sympathetic nervous system 24
symptoms and problems 60–70, *63*
  anorexia 69
  breathlessness 62–5
  cardiac pain 68–9
  constipation 69
  dry mouth 69–70
  fatigue 65–6, *66*
  nausea 69
  non-cardiac pain 66–8, *67*
  reported incidence 2–3, *3, 7*, 61
systolic ejection fraction indicators 51

Taylor, M and Ogden, J 98
team care 15, *16*, 111, 114–17, 126–7
teenagers 131
TENS 68
thalidomide 70
TNFα-blockers 26
Torbay palliative care services 141–2
training workshops, communication skills
  96–7
transplant issues 40, 41–2, 122–3

trazodone 78
treatment withdrawal
  consent issues 122
  patient requests 113–14, 115
trepopnoea 26
tricyclic antidepressants 63, 78
troponins 52

user involvement 132
Utrecht study (Bouvey *et al.*) 54–5, 55

VALIANT study 34
valsartan 34
venlafaxine 78
ventricular resynchronisation 25, 40
ventricular tachycardia 25
Viagra 129
vomiting 63, 69

warfarin 37
'warning shots' communication 95
weight loss 48–9

anorexia 69
Whiston Hospital (Liverpool) 140–1
withdrawal of treatments
  consent issues 122
  patient requests 113–14, 115

xerostomia 69–70

young people with heart failure 119–33
  care pathways 121–3
  end-of-life choices 131–2
  exercise and activity 125
  family and carer issues 127–8, 130–1
  funding support 126
  having children 129–30
  heart transplant issues 122–3
  participation in clinical trials 119–20
  physical needs and support 124–5, 126
  recognising mortality 123–4
  sexual needs 128–9
  teenagers and children 131
  timing of care 120–1